Clinical Use of Psychotherapeutic Drugs

Clinical Use of Psychotherapeutic Drugs

By

LEO E. HOLLISTER, M.D.

Medical Investigator
Veterans Administration Hospital
Associate Professor of Medicine
Stanford University
School of Medicine
Palo Alto, California

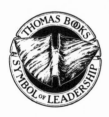

CHARLES C THOMAS ● PUBLISHER
SPRINGFIELD · ILLINOIS · U.S.A.

Published and Distributed Throughout the World by

CHARLES C THOMAS • PUBLISHER

Bannerstone House

301-327 East Lawrence Avenue, Springfield, Illinois, U.S.A.

© *1973, by* CHARLES C THOMAS • PUBLISHER

ISBN 0-398-02749-8

Library of Congress Catalog Card Number: 72-93214

PREFACE

ALMOST anyone who works in a field concludes, sooner or later, "I should write a book." This thought first occurred to me about a decade ago, after several years of clinical experience in the evaluation of psychotherapeutic drugs. Subsequently, a number of other books on psychotherapeutic drugs appeared, and this development, along with many other commitments of my own, allowed me to resist successfully this impulse until now.

Why write another book on the clinical use of psychotherapeutic drugs now? First, I was amazed to find while lecturing at various hospitals and teaching centers around the country how much clinicians and students desire both practical information about the use of these drugs as well as some concept of the scientific basis for their use. Second, the response to relatively brief review articles in medical journals was an overwhelming request for reprints, often in multiples, which also seemed to confirm a need. Finally, we have reached a plateau or consolidation phase in the history of psychotherapeutic drugs where radically new treatments (such as these drugs were only a little more than a decade ago) are not appearing. Much of our recent effort has been spent in trying to learn how better to use those drugs we have.

My purpose in this book has been to provide a general approach to drug therapy for mental and emotional disorders rather than a detailed description of individual drugs, doses, dosage schedules, formulations and all those bits and pieces of information which are so readily available in package inserts, the *Physicians Desk Reference,* or other sources. Rather than addressing myself to others who work in the field, so as to impress colleagues with my erudition, this book is directed to those clinical practitioners of psychiatry or other medical specialties who use these drugs in their clinical practice, and to students, who may find that the treatment of this large group of drugs leaves something to be desired in most textbooks of pharmacology. Some attempt has been made to justify the recommendations for use based on chemical and pharmacological principles, but no pretense is made that this work is a scholarly endeavor in those recondite areas.

As in any field, differences of opinion about the proper uses of these drugs abound. Any statement, if it is not banal, will also be contentious. The reader should be warned that these are personal opinions, which although based on long clinical and investigative experience, are not to go unchallenged. My major hope is that he may be spurred to compare them with his own experience and that of others, so that he may use these agents to their fullest potential for helping his patients.

LEO E. HOLLISTER

CONTENTS

Clinical Use of Psychotherapeutic Drugs

CHAPTER 1

INTRODUCTION

MENTAL illness may be both more frequent and more incapacitating than any other disease or disorder. Probably one-half of all visits to physicians are based on some emotional or mental disorder. Almost two million persons in the United States are at any given moment under some formal treatment for mental illness. An epidemological survey in midtown Manhattan led to the conclusion that only 20 percent of persons could be qualified as normal. While it must be devoutly hoped that Manhattan is not a model for the rest of the world, such a statistic is staggering (17).

Psychiatrists recognize many varieties of mental or emotional disorders (it is difficult to talk of "mental diseases" in the absence of a pathogenetic basis). Such a vast number of "therapies" abound that the situation was easily made the subject of parody a number of years ago (218). Each year some new therapy is announced, usually a rediscovery or renaming of a technique known before. To some extent the same situation applies to drug therapy, as in recent years, novelty in new drugs has been more likely to be the change of one atom for another in the structural formula. Drug therapy nonetheless has an important place in modern psychiatric treatment, but, like all other treatments can be harmful if done poorly.

HISTORICAL BACKGROUND

Kraepelin published an essay, "On the influence of several medicaments on simple psychic processes" in 1892, ten years after he had begun these investigations, and before his epochal achievement in dividing functional psychoses into two major divisions, dementia praecox and manic-depressive psychosis. Freud, too, was an early psychopharmacologist, having studied cocaine, among other drugs. He apparently thought that the solution to major mental disorders was more likely through chemical intervention than by psychoanalysis. Although these and other examples suggest that psychopharmacology is not an especially new discipline, the modern era began in the early 1950's. The first use of the word, "psychopharmacon" (from which "psychopharmacology" was derived), was in 1548 as the title of a prayer book for dying individuals (197).

Somatic therapies in psychiatry really began with the sequence leading to the treatment of dementia paralytica with drugs and physical methods. The introduction of arsphenamine as a treatment for syphilis, the proof of the syphilitic origin of general paresis, the amelioration of organic arsenical treatment by artificially induced fever (based on the fact that patients with paresis who survived typhus fever were improved), and finally the eradication of neurosyphilis by penicillin occurred over a 35-year period preceding modern psychotherapeutic drugs. Insulin shock, drug-induced seizures and finally electrically-induced convulsions date from the 1930's. Insulin shock, because of its great dangers and expense, was on the wane before the introduction of modern drugs. Electroconvulsive therapy has been largely supplanted by drug treatment, perhaps excessively so. Prefrontal leucotomy, another product of the 1930's, was eliminated by drugs, but much less destructive and more precise types of psychosurgery are once again being experimented with.

The first modern psychotherapeutic drug, lithium carbonate, dates from 1949, but through a variety of circumstances only became popular in recent years. Lithium was found to protect guinea pigs against toxic effects of urea, producing a state of lethargy which led to its experimental use in mania. Rauwolfia root was the subject of a number of reports since 1931 in the Indian medical literature, both as a treatment for hypertension and mania. Reserpine was isolated in 1952 by two chemists in the Ciba Laboratories in Basel and soon after was put to clinical use both in cardiology and psychiatry. Chlorpromazine was synthesized in 1950 at Rhone-Poulenc Laboratories in France, as part of a program to develop antihistaminic phenothiazine derivatives (110). It was first used in 1951, along with promethazine (another antihistaminic phenothiazine) and meperidine, as part of a "lytic cocktail" for a new type of anesthesia. It was noted that it had unusual sedative properties and in 1952 was first tested in France for the treatment of schizophrenic patients. The monoamine oxidase inhibitors had a checkered history, for sporadic trials in psychiatric patients followed the observation that iproniazid produced euphoria in patients with tuberculosis. Unfortunately, most of the trials were made with isoniazid, a better antituberculous drug but a relatively weak enzyme inhibitor. By 1952, the potent enzyme-inhibiting property of iproniazid had been described. As the importance of monoamines in the central nervous system and in the action mechanisms of other psychoactive drugs developed during the 1950s, it became inevitable that monoamine oxidase inhibitors would be tried clinically, as they were in 1957. The tricyclic antidepressants, because of their close resemblance chemically to the phenothiazines, were originally thought to be potential antipsychotic drugs. Only by the excellent clinical observation that imipramine was beneficial for depressed patients rather than schizophrenics was its antidepressant effect appreciated in 1957. A curious thread that weaves through the modern history of psychotherapeutic drugs is that most were initially planned for other uses and the psychiatric uses discovered more or less fortuitously in the clinic.

IMPACT OF MODERN PSYCHOTHERAPEUTIC DRUGS

Psychiatric thinking and practice were drastically altered by the introduction of these new psychotherapeutic drugs. One of the ways in which psychiatric thinking has changed is that one considers more and more likely the possibility that a great many "functional" psychiatric disorders have a genetic, and therefore biochemical, cause. Schizophrenia, that mysterious and crippling affliction, became both amenable to chemical treatment and possible to mimic, at least in some respects, by chemicals. The antipsychotic drugs have not cured schizophrenia, nor has the model psychosis from lysergic acid diethylamide (LSD-25) unraveled its biochemical basis. Still, we think more of genes and amines in seeking to explain schizophrenia than we do of dreams and schemes of the unconscious (94). The case for a biochemical substrate of serious mental depressions is even more advanced. These disorders also seem to have a pattern of genetic transmission, and the ability to produce a model of them in man, by reserpine, as well as the elucidation of the mode of action of some of the antidepressant drugs, has evolved into the "amine hypothesis" of depression (43, 75). That the pendulum should swing back towards a new emphasis on biological psychiatry is not surprising. After all, the only major psychiatric disorder to be eliminated in the present century, general paresis due to syphilis, yielded to techniques of the biological sciences.

The hospital practice of psychiatry has changed remarkably in the past two decades. Before the advent of modern drugs, one of every two hospital beds in the United States was occupied by a psychiatric patient, fully 50 percent of these by victims of schizophrenia. Since 1955, when these drugs first had widespread clinical impact, the number of hospital beds occupied by psychiatric patients has steadily declined. Some hospitals have only one-quarter to one-tenth the bed occupancy of fifteen years ago. Proposals have been made to eliminate many mental hospitals and to transfer almost entirely the care of mentally ill patients to the community. Such trends would have been unthinkable without the availability of drugs which curb the deteriorating course of serious mental disorders. Unfortunately, good as drugs have been they are not good enough. We have many patients who are better and too few who are well.

Aside from changes in numbers of patients in mental hospitals, the hospitals themselves underwent remarkable changes. From being prisons, they became true hospitals, with locked wards either completely disappearing or being only reserved for the most seriously disturbed patients for brief periods of time. The rights of patients to personal belongings, to a voice in the conduct of their treatment, and to escape from involuntary confinement were accelerated, if not made possible, by the advent of effective drug therapy. Hospital personnel who used to devote most of their energies to custodial duties have now all become "therapists." While much of what passes for "psychotherapy" may be intuitively based, the assertion that persons with no medical training and relatively little experience can manage drugs effectively is dangerous nonsense; amateur drug therapists can be disastrous.

NOMENCLATURE OF PSYCHOTHERAPEUTIC DRUGS

The initial epithet "tranquilizer" was devised because "sedative" had become a dirty word among psychiatrists after the belated discovery that barbiturates might lead to physical dependence. The implications of the two words are the same, so that widespread adoption of the term "tranquilizer" implied that drugs so labeled were really newer types of sedatives. To some extent this was true, especially in regard to the antianxiety drugs, but in the case of phenothiazine derivatives and other antipsychotics, the confusion caused by the inappropriate term is still widespread. One still hears them referred to as "chemical straitjackets" despite the abundant evidence that they are liberating rather than constricting agents. Attempts have been made to differentiate "tranquilizers" from conventional sedatives by introducing the divisions, "major" and "minor," or by coining Greek-root neologisms such as "ataractic," "neuroleptic," "psycholeptic" or "psychoinhibitor." These terms, too, suffered from some implicit assumptions about the modes of action of drugs so labeled. By the same token, one had for so long associated an "antidepressant" drug with a stimulant that even today tricyclic antidepressants are often referred to as stimulants, something they clearly are not.

A more realistic nomenclature might be based on the putative clinical uses of the various drugs. Drugs used for treating anxiety, in all its many clinical guises, would be referred to as antianxiety drugs; those for mental depressions, as antidepressants; and those used for treating schizophrenia and other psychoses would be termed antipsychotic drugs. With the advent of drugs for treating mania, one can speak of antimanic drugs. Even such a nomenclature has defects; each of the drug types may, under certain circumstances, be used for the other purposes. Nonetheless, the "anti-" system of nomenclature has greater simplicity and more clinical relevance than any of the others.

SPECIAL PROBLEMS IN EVALUATING
PSYCHOTHERAPEUTIC AGENTS

Uncertain Diagnoses and Pathogenesis

Psychiatric diagnosis is almost completely based on inference. With the exception of those acute and chronic brain syndromes associated with neuropathological abnormalities, most psychiatric disorders leave none of the visible marks which provide confirmatory feed-back from the necropsy room. The data upon which we make our inferences are soft, being based on what patients tell us, what we infer from what they tell or how they act, or what other people tell us about them. Even the most precise psychological testing makes only the grossest sort of distinctions, such as a "functional" rather than an "organic" disorder.

Despite these difficulties, clinical data of the type mentioned can at least be handled in a standardized fashion. Psychometric codification of these data and criteria for their evaluation can be developed to permit a semiquantitative appraisal of the degree of departure from normal as well as a qualitative profile of the type of psychopathology present. Numerous psychiatric rating scales have been developed to assess most psychiatric disorders in some such "objective" way, especially since the advent of psychotherapeutic drugs. Experience with these methods indicates that psychometric assessments approach the validity and the level of consensual agreement between raters that one might expect from interpretations of abnormal electrocardiograms or chest x-rays.

Not only do we lack the ability to verify diagnosis by the ultimate demonstration of some pathological change, but we have little concept of the pathogenesis of the illnesses we are treating. Theories of pathogenesis for the functional psychiatric disorders abound, but evidence for any of these is relatively scanty. Nosologic nomenclature has become the refuge of our ignorance. At times, frustration with psychiatric nomenclature has led to the suggestion that all psychiatric diagnosis be abandoned and that patients be described in terms of disturbances in psychodynamics. To many, this suggestion is analogous to substituting the intangible for the nebulous. Recently, the tendency has been to classify empirical groupings of psychiatric disorders based on the presenting clinical symptoms and signs and demographic variables in patients (143, 169). Such groupings have verified the major traditional diagnostic categories of psychiatric patients but have decreased the subdivisions. They appear to have some value in differentiating between responses to drugs. Still, it is highly doubtful that such empirical classifications will add to our basic understanding of the various functional psychiatric disorders.

Confounding Variables

Due to uncertainty regarding pathogenesis, multifaceted treatment programs are used with most emotional disorders. The old adage that the lack of a single effective treatment encourages multiple treatments is nowhere more evident. The number of "therapies" offered psychiatric patients continues to multiply. While no one could argue against any measures which may help patients, it is obvious that the many treatments offered confound the problem of drug effects to varying degrees.

Controlled Clinical Trials

Besides the influence of concurrent treatments, the course of many emotional disorders is variable, with some spontaneous improvement or remission. Not every anxious patient is always so; environmental influences play a considerable role in determining the degree of anxiety. The same is true of depression, a fact which has been documented repeatedly during controlled studies of antidepressant drugs. Schizophrenic reactions also may remit spontaneously, although apparently not as often as thought. They may also become worse in the absence of effective treatment.

To control for these extrinsic variables, controlled clinical trials have been used extensively for evaluating psychotherapeutic drugs. Such trials are based on large, homogeneous samples of patients, random assignments of treatments, blind controls, objective recording, and statistical analysis of data. Although none of these techniques was initiated by clinical psychopharmacologists, it is fair to say that they reached full flower in the study of psychotherapeutic drugs.

One should not be dogmatic about controlled trials. Valid observations can be made by good clinicians in the absence of formal controls; premature controlled studies may even be misleading. They are to be done only after the proper indications, dose, and most common side effects of a drug are known. Finally, it should be realized that controlled studies scarcely ever reveal a new treatment, but simply confirm or deny expectations about a drug. In making clinical judgments about the effectiveness of drugs as therapy, however, evidence from controlled studies should be given greatest weight.

OVER- OR UNDER-USE

Psychotherapeutic drugs accounted for 17 percent of all prescriptions in a survey of drug use in an American community. "Tranquilizers" accounted for 7.7 percent of all prescriptions, hypnotics and sedatives for 3.6 percent and amphetamines for 3.4 percent, the latter being the eighth in rank of frequently prescribed drugs (221). Such surveys only tap the use of psychotherapeutic drugs in the private sector of medicine. As most hospital care of mental disorders is done by the public sector, the percentage for the latter would very likely be much higher. No one can argue that these drugs are not widely used.

The argument seems to center about whether or not they are wisely used. On the one hand are those who directly accuse the pharmaceutical companies of "mystifying" the indications for their drugs, by means of promotional material suggesting use of drugs to relieve trivial symptoms (140). For instance, an antianxiety drug was promoted for treating the anxiety children suffer when they first leave their families to go away to school. Such anxiety is obviously better worked through rather than relieved by the artifice of drugs. Implicit in such accusations are that physicians are easily gulled by such advertisements. Such an assertion is by no means established (in fact it may be questioned how many of these advertisements are actually read) but is easily made. Others, whose bias is clear from the pejorative term "over-medicated society" in the title of their paper, suggest that physicians are not just stupid, but rather lazy (161). They prescribe psychotherapeutic drugs because they don't want to take the time to deal with patients. Kafka put it much better: "Writing prescriptions is easy; understanding patients is difficult." Of course, one assumes that given a proper amount of time, a physician (or more likely some "therapist" of varied credentials) would be able to deal with the patient in such a way that drugs would not be needed, again an assertion which lacks genuine proof.

On the other hand, data from a survey of drug use in California adults suggests that perhaps drugs are being used rather wisely. Although 50 percent of persons have used some psychotherapeutic drug during their lifetime, and 30 percent within the past year, frequent use occurs in only about 17 percent of adults. Women use drugs more than men (the latter no doubt using the social drug, alcohol, in lieu of prescribed drugs), and those whose supports in the form of religion (no affiliation) or family (divorced or separated) are lacking tend to use them the most. The patterns of frequent drug use change with age, stimulants being used by men in the 30's, tranquilizers in the 40's and 50's and sedatives in the 60's. Such data suggest that despite such frequent use of these drugs, they are used selectively and with some apparent rationale (149).

A small minority insist that drugs are under-used, that many patients suffer needlessly because physicians have become so fearful of creating drug dependent individuals that they use drugs less often than required. While such a situation may happen occasionally, it is doubtful that it is the rule. Nonetheless, physicians can be moved to strange positions by prevailing public opinion. Witness the absurd situation in regard to amphetamines. Physicians are now eagerly confessing that for over thirty years they employed a group of drugs with no therapeutic use. Why? Because some clucks have taken the same drug and have given it to themselves intravenously in 10 to 100 times the usual oral doses used for treatment and have had some harmful effects from this practice. Had aspirin been abused in a similar fashion, the results would have been far more devastating. But would it make sense to deny the efficacy of aspirin because of such abuse?

Extreme positions are rarely valid. The proper use of psychotherapeutic drugs is not to be measured by how many people use them, or how often, but under what circumstances and with what effects. The prudent use of psychotherapeutic drugs demands the same skills required for the use of any other type of drug: proper diagnosis, proper selection of drug, proper doses and dosage schedules, and careful clinical followup. If these conditions are met, one need not worry about whether patients are getting too much or too few of these drugs.

DESIDERATA

The ideal psychotherapeutic drug would: (a) cure or alleviate the pathogenetic mechanisms of the symptom or disorder; (b) be rapidly effective; (c) benefit most or all patients for whom it is indicated; (d) be nonhabituating and lack potential for creating dependence; (e) not have tolerance develop; (f) have minimum toxicity on the therapeutic range; (g) have a low incidence of secondary side effects; (h) would not be lethal in overdoses; (i) be adaptable both to inpatients and outpatients; and (j) not impair any cognitive, perceptual or motor functions. No such drug exists, but to a fairly surprising degree many of the available drugs meet the majority of these desiderata. It has been both our blessing and our curse that we had effective drug therapy for emotional disorders before we had a science of behavioral pathology. Our best hope for getting better psychotherapeutic drugs is to understand better the causes of emotional disorders.

CHAPTER 2

ANTIPSYCHOTIC DRUGS

FEW illnesses compare with schizophrenia in taking such a toll of the most useful years of an individual's life. Few illnesses have been so frustrating to explain or treat. Few illnesses create such sadness and guilt in those who cannot find ways to help their affected loved one. "Cures" are rare indeed; probably less than 15 percent of individuals seriously affected who require any kind of prolonged hospitalization ever again function "normally." Schizophrenia and alcoholism are the two major problems in psychiatry; they deserve far more attention than they have been given in the past.

Although the disaster that is schizophrenia has been partially mitigated by drugs, our knowledge of the pathophysiological mechanisms of this disorder is still meager. The impetus provided by the success of drugs in treating this disorder resulted in many inquiries into the biological bases for it (228). Older notions that schizophrenia is a reaction to social-psychological influences, such as that it represents a disordered learning process initiated and sustained by conflicting messages from mother, have few remaining adherents. The present tendency is to regard schizophrenia as a genetically determined disorder with biological mechanisms whose phenotypic expression may be influenced in part by life experiences. As antischizophrenic drugs were discovered fortuitously, our continuing lack of knowledge of the pathogenesis of the disorder has limited development of more effective drugs. We have new chemicals, but old drugs.

The term "antipsychotic" drug should in no way imply that these drugs are curative. Rather one might consider them analogous to bacteriostatic as contrasted with bacterial antibiotics. They may simply relieve secondary symptoms of schizophrenia and arrest or ameliorate the natural course of the disorder. Even should these drugs prove ultimately to have provided no more

13

than symptomatic relief, they should not be denigrated. Most treatment in medicine is symptomatic, despite our desires to think the contrary.

CHEMICAL AND PHARMACOLOGICAL DIFFERENCES

At present, nine chemical classes of compounds are known which ameliorate psychoses and evoke extrapyramidal reactions, the two unique properties of antipsychotic drugs. The three classes currently in use in the United States are shown in Figure 2-1. Although some close resemblances between the chemical structures of the phenothiazines and thioxanthenes are apparent, resemblances between these types of drugs and the butyro-phenones are less obvious.

The structures of most antipsychotic drugs can be viewed as tertiary or rarely, secondary, amines derived from methylethyl-amine (-C-C-N-C). Phenothiazine antipsychotics have the following common S-shaped configuration, regardless of which subfamily they belong to (R-N-C-C-C-N-C). The thioxanthenes show a similar

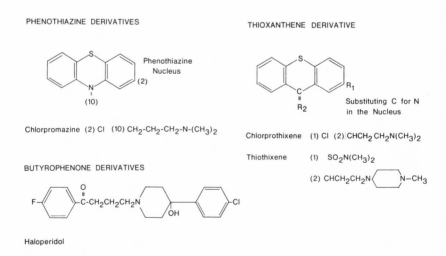

Figure 2-1. Structures of the three classes of antipsychotic drugs available in the United States.

nucleus (R-C-C-C-C-N-C), as do the butyrophenones (R-C-C-C-C-N-C). This conformation of the molecule may be critical to its effect (116, 217). On the other hand, the side chain substituents which show this conformation are not specific to antipsychotic drugs, as similar configurations can be found among some of the tricyclic antidepressants. Here the major difference may be in the planarity of the molecule, the phenothiazines being coplanar while the tricyclics are not.

The phenothiazine derivatives are the longest known and most popular antipsychotics. Partly because of chemical differences but also because of variations in pharmacological actions and potency, distinction between the three chemical subfamilies of phenothiazines should be made (Fig. 2-2). Compounds with an aliphatic dimethylaminopropyl side-chain, such as chlorpromazine, are relatively low in potency and high in sedative effects. Substitution at the 2-position of the phenothiazine nucleus creates a more potent compound than no substitution; for example, chlorpromazine is more potent than promazine. Some substituents such as the trifluoromethyl group confer more potency than a simple chlorine atom (triflupromazine is more potent than chlorpromazine). The nuclear substituents may increase potency by increasing fat solubility of the molecule. The piperidine side-chain is represented by thioridazine and its side-chain sulfoxide metabolite, mesoridazine, both most different from other phenothiazines in pharmacological actions. Piperacetazine, technically a piperidinyl phenothiazine, has pharmacological properties which are more like those of the piperazine group, to which it has a closer spatial configuration. Three variants of the piperazine side-chain, along with variations of the ring substituent, create a rather large class of piperazinyl phenothiazines. These compounds are much more potent than their ring-substituted analogs in the aliphatic series. They tend to possess less sedative effects than the other two classes, but are more likely to produce extrapyramidal reactions at equivalent therapeutic doses.

The relationship between the thioxanthenes and the phenothiazines is clearly evident (See Fig. 2-1). Substitution of the carbon-atom for the nitrogen-atom in the ring alters the geometry of the molecule somewhat. Chlorprothixene is the thioxanthene

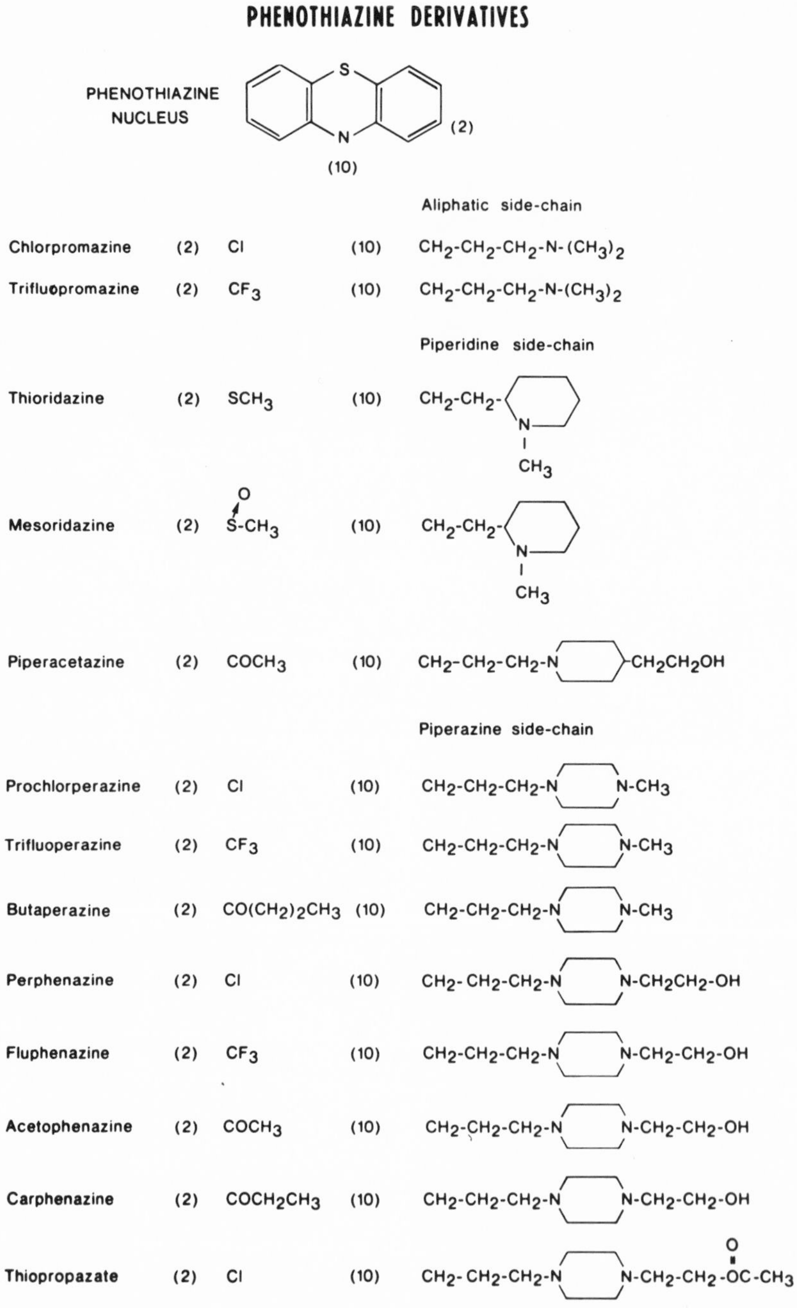

PHENOTHIAZINE DERIVATIVES

Figure 2-2. Various members of the three subfamilies of phenothiazine derivatives.

analog of chlorpromazine, while thiothixene is the analog of the very potent phenothiazine, thioproperazine. The combination of the unique dimethylsulfonamide ring substituent, as well as the piperazine side-chain of thiothixene makes for a more potent compound, although in general the thioxanthenes are somewhat less potent than their phenothiazine homologs.

The chemical structure of haloperidol is typical for butyrophenones. Virtually all the variations in structure have involved portions of the phenylpiperidine moiety, sometimes being simply ring substituents of differing types, sometimes involving formation of a single piperazine ring or two piperidine rings, but never disturbing the position of the nitrogen in the piperidine ring (Fig. 2-3). In the case of trifluperidol, an analog studied several years ago, the only difference from haloperidol was a shift in location and type of the halogen substituent on the phenyl ring. Although technically not a butyrophenone, pimozide is clearly derived from the same type of structure. More recently a number of diphenylbutylpiperidines have evolved from this group. Some of these, such as fluspirilene and penfluridol, are extremely long-acting compounds when given orally (226).

Aliphatic and piperidinyl phenothiazines tend to be "high-dose" drugs with doses measured in 100's of mg per day as compared with piperizinyl phenothiazines, the more potent thioxanthenes and butyrophenones. The latter are considered "low-dose" drugs with daily doses in the 10's of mg. Potency should never be confused with efficacy, as despite their greater potency, low-dose drugs offer no advantages in terms of total efficacy. They do offer a generally higher ratio between the desired antipsychotic effects and other undesired pharmacological effects such as sedation and alpha adrenergic blocking action. The French phrase for such a drug is "neuroleptique incisif," the English equivalent being "a more specific antipsychotic drug."

Several other chemical classes have antipsychotic activity, but for various reasons these drugs are not used in the United States (Fig. 2-4). The Rauwolfia alkaloids have become obsolete, although reserpine was widely used early on and is still a most interesting pharmacological tool. Some resemblance to the chemical structure or reserpine can be seen in the benzoquinolizines, although the latter lack the indole configuration.

Benzquinamide, a benzoquinolizine derivative, despite the fact that it has definite antipsychotic effects, will not be introduced into the American market for this purpose but rather as an antiemetic. Oxypertine is only one of a large number of phenylpiperazine derivatives which range over a broad spectrum of psychotherapeutic activity. This drug is more widely used for anxiety and depression elsewhere in the world than it is used as an antipsychotic. Another compound with an indolic structure, molindone, has definite antipsychotic action, but it still has not

BUTYROPHENONES AND RELATED COMPOUNDS

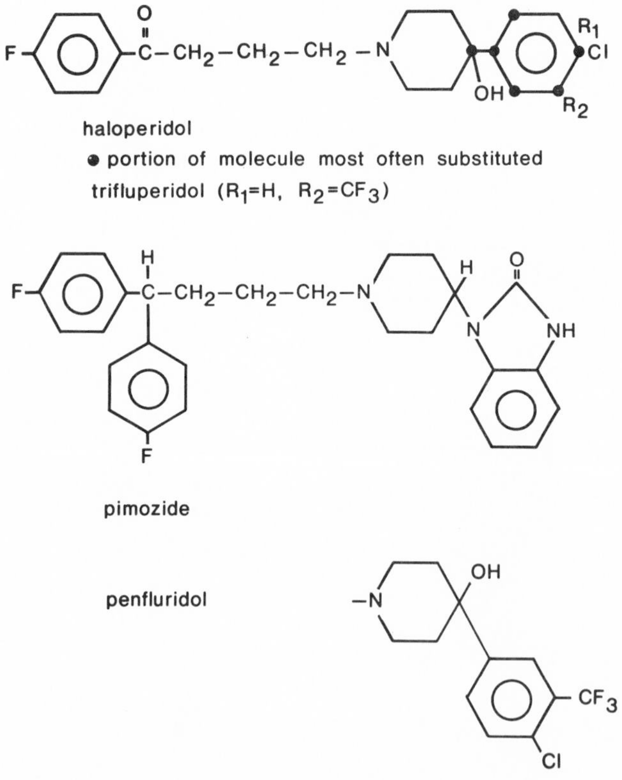

haloperidol

● portion of molecule most often substituted
trifluperidol (R$_1$=H, R$_2$=CF$_3$)

pimozide

penfluridol

Figure 2-3. Relationships between the butyrophenones and some diphenyl-butylpiperidine derivatives.

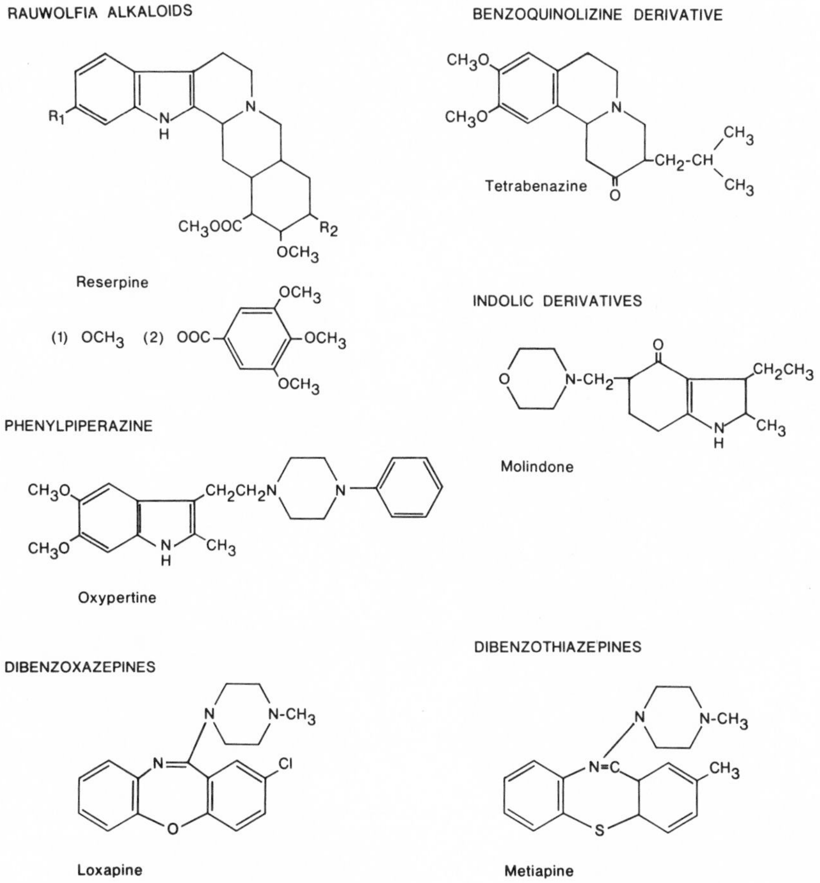

RAUWOLFIA ALKALOIDS

BENZOQUINOLIZINE DERIVATIVE

Tetrabenazine

Reserpine

(1) OCH₃ (2) OOC

PHENYLPIPERAZINE

INDOLIC DERIVATIVES

Molindone

Oxypertine

DIBENZOXAZEPINES

DIBENZOTHIAZEPINES

Loxapine

Metiapine

Figure 2-4. Structures of chemical classes of antipsychotic drugs either not sold in the United States or still in investigational status.

reached the market, presumably because it offers no special advantage over other drugs currently available. Two related new classes of drugs, the dibenzoxazepines and the dibenzothiazepines, are currently under clinical trials, but seem to be active as antipsychotics.

COMMON PHARMACOLOGICAL PROPERTIES

All antipsychotic drugs share two novel pharmacological actions which were unknown prior to their advent: (a) the ability to ameliorate the course of schizophrenia and (b) the ability to evoke in many patients extrapyramidal syndromes of various types, including one that mimics strongly naturally-occurring Parkinson's disease. For a long while it was uncertain why these two unusual and seemingly unrelated effects should be linked. Now it appears that both are mediated through the same biochemical mechanism, decreased dopaminergic transmission in those pathways in the brain that use this neurotransmitter. The case for the involvement of dopamine in Parkinson syndromes has been strongly supported by the use of its precursor, levodopa, as a treatment for Parkinson's disease. The case for the same involvement of dopamine in schizophrenia is far less secure. One would have to postulate two somewhat distinct dopaminergic pathways, one dealing with mental effects (amelioration of schizophrenia) and one with motor effects (evocation of extrapyramidal syndromes).

The term "neuroleptic action" implies four anatomical sites of action:
(1) at the reticular activating system of the midbrain, where sensory input is monitored;
(2) at the amygdala and hippocampus, structures in the limbic system that provide the emotional coloring attached to incoming signals;
(3) at the hypothalamus, which governs the peripheral responses to meaningful sensory information, by means both of the pituitary-endocrine system and the automonic nervous system;
(4) at the globus pallidus and corpus straitum, where extrapyramidal syndromes are elicited, perhaps coincidentally.

It can be appreciated that these drugs affect the function of the three major integrating systems of the brain, the reticular activating system, the limbic system and the hypothalamus. One might speculate that they could reduce extraneous or distracting sensory information, reduce the affective charge of all sensations, and reduce the somatic responses to them.

Attempts to relate the potency of drugs in producing extrapyramidal effects to their clinical efficacy or the development of extrapyramidal reactions in patients to their ultimate outcome have not been very rewarding. Some drugs which are rather potent in producing extrapyramidal reactions, such as reserpine, are not considered to be as efficacious for schizophrenia as others which are rather weak, such as thioridazine. In part, it may be due to a difference in mechanism; reserpine produces extrapyramidal reactions (and very likely its antipsychotic effects) by depleting the storage of dopamine and other biogenic amines in storage granules at the nerve ending rather than by blocking access of the neurotransmitter to its receptor. Thioridazine may be relatively weak in eliciting extrapyramidal reactions because its anticholinergic effects may be greater than other phenothiazines. All phenothiazines are weakly anticholinergic and it may be this action which allows their use at monumental doses without the production of extrapyramidal side effects (195).

All antipsychotics are sedative, which led to the erroneous term "tranquilizer." Although some have a reputation clinically as "activating" drugs, they are by no means stimulants. Rather, this reputation is based on an increased motor activity as well as a lesser sedative to antipsychotic ratio. Most are alpha adrenergic blocking drugs; some, such as chlorpromazine and thioridazine, being especially so. With the conspicuous exception of thioridazine, all are antiemetic drugs, which provides an additional clinical use. This latter coincidental pharmacological action led to the paradox that for many years the animal pharmacological test which correlated most highly with antipsychotic activity was the prevention of apomorphine-induced emesis in dogs. Surely this test was a most irrelevant model of schizophrenia in man.

Some of the postulated mechanisms of the antipsychotic effects of these drugs are shown in Table 2-I, indicating both specific and generalized loci of action.

Table 2-I

Postulated Bases of Antipsychotic Effects

post-synaptic block of noradrenergic or dopaminergic receptors

interaction with neuronal membrane to decrease exciteability (biophysical)

metabolic inhibition of oxidative phosphorylation, altering ionic pumps and decreasing neuronal excitability (biochemical)

PHARMACOLOGICAL SCREENING TESTS

It is perhaps unfortunate that antipsychotic drugs were first discovered in the clinic. Pharmacologists subsequently determined their effects in laboratory animals. From these studies have emerged a great many of the attributes of known antipsychotic drugs. These in turn are used to screen new chemical compounds for possible antipsychotic activity. One can see that this is a circular pathway, leading to an increasing number of compounds which may differ chemically but which are essentially similar pharmacologically. As yet no one has found a way to break out of this circular trap.

Some of the more predictive animal pharmacological screening tests for drugs with clinical antipsychotic activity are: (a) reduction of exploratory behavior without undue sedation; (b) induction of a cataleptic state; (c) induction of palpebral ptosis reversible through handling; (d) inhibition of conditioned avoidance behavior; (e) inhibition of intracranial self-stimulation reward areas; (f) inhibition of amphetamine- or apomorphine-induced stereotypic behaviors; (g) protection against epinephrine- or norepinephrine-induced mortality. One can easily see that most of these tests are only tangentially related, if at all, to the clinical manifestations of schizophrenia.

METABOLISM AND KINETICS OF CHLORPROMAZINE

Nearly all antipsychotic drugs are highly surface-active, lipophilic and weakly basic. Such physicochemical properties would favor accumulation in the brain and other tissues. The metabolism and kinetics of chlorpromazine has been most extensively studied, both because it was the prototypic drug as well as because of the substantial doses used, making measurement in biological fluids and tissues easier.

Although several technical methods have been proposed for measuring chlorpromazine and its metabolites in plasma, it is still not certain that they are reliable (224). Many of the inferences made from studies of plasma concentrations of drug or metabolites must be highly tentative. It is fairly easy to measure urinary metabolites of the drug, but the relevance of excretory patterns in the urine to concentrations in plasma or tissues, or to clinical effects, seems to be increasingly remote.

Chlorpromazine is almost completely absorbed, but it may be destroyed or metabolized to a variable extent as it passes through the intestinal wall (49). It is also fairly quickly metabolized in the liver, so that its metabolism is extensive. Some years ago, based on the then known pathways of metabolism, it was estimated that 168 metabolites were possible. Since the advent of combined gas-liquid chromatography and mass spectroscopy, many of these postulated metabolites have been identified (90). A simplified schema of the possible metabolic pathways of chlorpromazine is shown in Figure 2-5. Some metabolites have very little pharmacological activity, such as chlorpromazine sulfoxide, while others, such as 7-hydroxy-chlorpromazine seem to have a relatively high level of activity. Thus, it is still uncertain whether the major action of the drug is mediated by the parent compound or one or more active metabolites. The prolonged therapeutic benefits which may persist after withdrawal of the drug does little to settle the issue.

The drug is strongly bound to protein, which has contributed to much of the difficulty in measuring plasma concentrations. It is apparently concentrated in brain against a plasma gradient, reaching an estimated five-fold concentration in the brain of humans as compared with plasma concentrations. Only one study has been published on the tissue distribution of the drug in man. The lung has a very high concentration as do the keratin structures, such as the nails and hair. Distribution within the brain is uneven (67).

ROUTES OF METABOLISM OF CHLORPROMAZINE

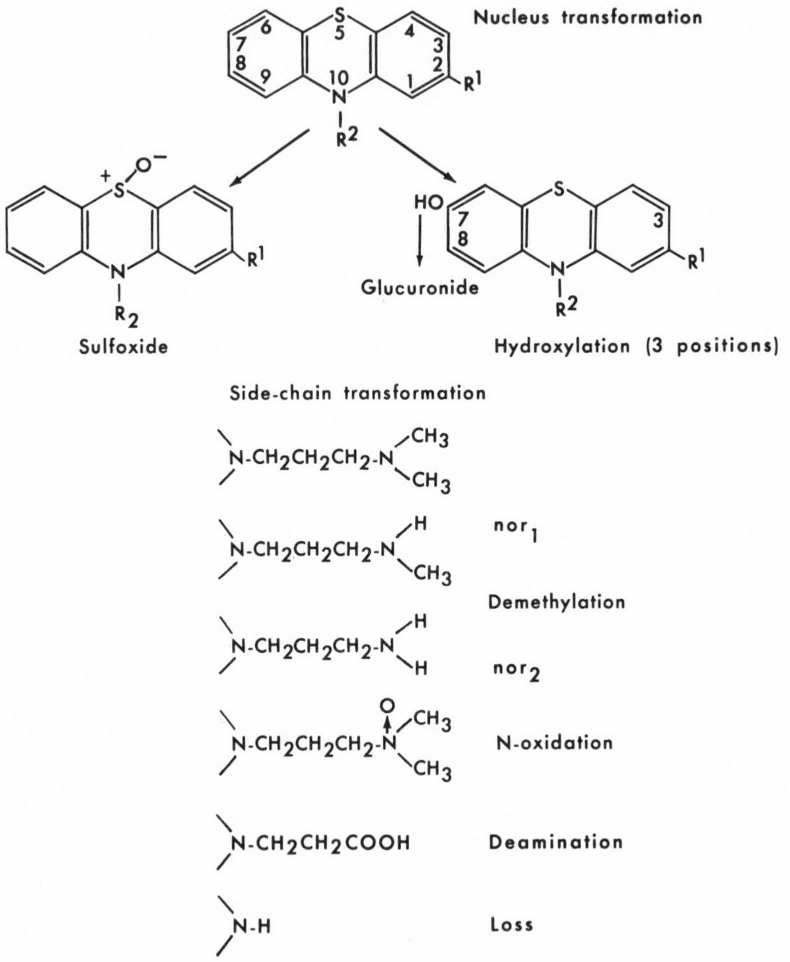

Figure 2-5. Schema of metabolism of chlorpromazine. Demethylation, hydroxylation and sulfoxidation are main routes. Activity of many metabolites remains undetermined.

Despite the difficulties in measuring plasma concentrations of the drug, some tentative conclusions may be reached. Following intramuscular administration of drug, a very rapid peak level is reached and drug never fails to be absorbed. Following oral doses, peak blood levels occur within 1½ to 3 hours, but absorption is sometimes very poor (107). When steady-state conditions have been reached, there are variations around successive dosings. The plasma half-life of chlorpromazine itself is short, being less than six hours in most subjects. This finding suggests either rapid metabolism or redistribution to tissues. As has generally been the case with psychoactive drugs, vast differences in steady-state plasma concentrations occur between different patients treated with similar daily doses of drug. It has been suggested that an optimal therapeutic level of drug in plasma lies between 25 and 300 ng/ml, with levels lower or higher than these leading to poor clinical responses (48). On the other hand, another group has not been able to establish any clear relationship between plasma levels of drug and clinical effects (56).

Urinary excretion of metabolites accounts for less than one-third the administered single dose over a 24-hour period. Conjugated metabolites account for about 69 percent of metabolites following oral doses and 87 percent after intramuscular doses. Within individuals in steady-state conditions, the proportion of conjugated metabolites remained rather constant, nor was there any tendency for increase with continued exposure to the drug (108). Nonetheless, it is possible that chlorpromazine may induce its own metabolizing enzymes. Even after discontinuation of chronic treatment, most patients continue to excrete chlorpromazine metabolites for about three months, although the range is from six weeks to six months (68).

The progress that has been made in understanding the metabolism and kinetics of chlorpromazine has been gratifying. Unfortunately, at present there are no reliable laboratory measurements that can be used to guide the clinician to a more effective use of the drug.

INDICATIONS FOR ANTIPSYCHOTIC DRUGS

Schizophrenia

Unique prejudices against drug therapy of schizophrenia existed when antipsychotic drugs were first introduced. The subsequent attempts to prove their efficacy in this disorder probably represent the most massive scientific overkill in clinical pharmacology. Large-scale cooperative controlled clinical trials involving thousands of patients were mounted by several groups to prove these drugs (2, 30, 31, 135, 157, 162). In virtually all studies, results were clear: Antipsychotic drugs were far more effective than placebo or ineffective drugs, such as barbiturates, and these favorable results were obtained at any stage of the illness, at any age of life, in either sex, at any place of treatment and with or without other interventions.

Over the course of years, it became apparent that many drugs were essentially equal in terms of overall efficacy. Thus, a large group of "peer" drugs were available from which the clinician could choose with reasonable assurance (See Table 2-II). Early on, it became apparent that the phenothiazines were more effective antipsychotics than was reserpine, a conclusion later supported by

Table 2-II

Antipsychotic Drugs Evaluated in
VA Collaborative Studies

Approximately equally effective:

chlorpromazine	thioridazine
prochlorperazine	fluphenazine
triflupromazine	acetophenazine
perphenazine	thiopropazate
haloperidol	thiothixene
trifluperidol	chlorprothixene
benzquinamide	oxypertine

Less effective than above:

promazine	reserpine
mepazine	molindone

several controlled studies. As a consequence, reserpine has lapsed into virtual disuse as an antipsychotic drug. Mepazine and promazine, the two phenothiazines which seemed to be less effective than the others, have suffered somewhat similar fates; the former drug was withdrawn from the market, as much for its toxicity as its inefficacy, and the latter is scarcely used for prolonged treatment. Evidence for the efficacy of the newer classes of antipsychotics is less impressive than for the phenothiazines, but enough to be convincing. Chlorprothixene and thiothixene, the two thioxanthene derivatives, have each been shown to rank with the effective phenothiazines in newly admitted patients. The same is true for haloperidol, the sole available butyrophenone, which was equal to thiopropazate in a controlled study. Benzquinamide, a benzoquinolizine derivative which was never marketed, also appeared to be as effective as perphenazine or acetophenazine under the conditions of a controlled trial. Trials with oxypertine, a still experimental drug, indicate its efficacy in certain types of schizophrenics. Early studies of molindone also reveal some degree of antipsychotic activity.

The impressive efficacy of antipsychotic drugs for an illness which had seemed to respond only to the whims of fate clearly established drug therapy as the primary treatment of schizophrenics. In fact, it became increasingly apparent from the many controlled studies that drug therapy was the only one whose ameliorative effects could be definitely distinguished. After some initial restriction of other "therapies" as possible confounding variables, it became customary to evaluate drugs within the context of a full hospital treatment program. Under such conditions, patients treated with effective antipsychotics improved, while those who received ineffective drugs or placebos were little changed. This does not mean that none of the latter patients improved, but rather that each improved patient was offset by one who became worse, while the majority were unchanged. Not all patients treated with antipsychotic drugs are helped. Many who are helped still leave much to be desired. We need better drugs than we have, good as they are.

Another fact soon became apparent. The benefits from

antipsychotics were not due simply to sedation. Rather, many prominent symptoms of schizophrenia which had failed previously to respond to sedatives were ameliorated. Disturbed thinking, paranoid symptoms, delusions, emotional and social withdrawal, and personal neglect improved as well as anxiety and agitation, symptoms which might be expected to respond to conventional sedatives. Regardless of the how it was accomplished, the alleviation of such characteristic psychotic symptoms by these drugs justified the epithet "antipsychotic."

Improvement from drugs approximates the familiar learning curve. There is rapid change in the first few weeks, a slowing of improvement in the 6th to 12th weeks of treatment, and very slow change thereafter. There is often an unevenness in rate of symptom change; hyperactivity may disappear after only a few doses of a phenothiazine, while delusions and hallucinations may persist, with lessened affect, for weeks. Abnormal thinking and interpersonal relationships in catatonic patients may improve weeks before the pathologic motor pattern is altered. Changes for the better are more apt to occur in women than in men.

The effects of drug therapy on the natural course of schizophrenia remain unknown; it may never be possible to determine them. Few good studies were done prior to the drug era. So many other treatment modalities have since been introduced that all results are confounded. One would have supposed that prompt treatment of the acutely ill patient with an adequate drug would produce a more lasting result than deferred treatment. Yet, a followup study of a group of acutely ill patients treated for the first 12 weeks of hospitalization either with phenobarbital or with one of five phenothiazines, indicated that over a 3-year period the patients initially treated with phenobarbital (later treated, of course, with antipsychotics) had about the same course as the others in regard to rates of discharge and readmission. Early treatment with drugs may not be so important as once postulated.

Other Functional Psychoses

Phenothiazine derivatives and butyrophenones control the

symptoms of manic reactions quickly and fairly completely. Since
the introduction in 1949 of lithium carbonate as a treatment,
interest in this novel approach has steadily grown. Its use will be
discussed further in Chapter 3. As will also be seen, depressive
syndromes accompanied by a large component of agitation may be
improved with a phenothiazine or a thioxanthene. Psychotic
paranoid reactions treated with higher dosage ranges of antipsychotic drugs for fairly extended periods may become stabilized
and show lessening of tension level and agitation.

Organic Brain Syndromes

Patients with chronic brain syndromes of any etiology who are
overactive and delusional often respond well to phenothiazine
compounds used cautiously in small doses. Though seizures may
sometimes be precipitated, phenothiazines have been used in
management of behavioral disturbances in chronic epileptics.
However, the benzodiazepines are more logical choices as they also
have anticonvulsant properties. Etiology in acute brain syndromes
is a more important consideration since some delirious states stem
from physiologic disturbances which could be aggravated by the
phenothiazines. Phenothiazines and butyrophenones, though often
used for treating withdrawal reactions from alcohol and other
drugs, can no longer be considered as appropriate for these
conditions (120). The basic principle of treating with pharmacologically equivalent drugs still holds, and the use of conventional
sedatives such as pentobarbital sodium or chlordiazepoxide, for
treating alcohol withdrawal or the use of opioids such as
methadone, for treating withdrawal from the opium derivatives is
still to be greatly preferred (see Chapter 7).

PRINCIPLES IN THE USE OF ANTIPSYCHOTIC DRUGS

No Trivial Indications

The indications for antipsychotic drugs discussed above are all
major psychiatric illnesses. Had chlorpromazine not been so
effective in a previously untreatable disorder, its extensive toxicity

might have prevented its clinical acceptance. All antipsychotics are potent and sometimes toxic drugs. They should be used for what they do best, and not for uses that other drugs may do equally or better.

Antipsychotic drugs are sometimes given in large parenteral doses to curb nonschizophrenic excitement, as for instance, a "bad trip" from some hallucinogenic drug. Management of such acutely agitated or excited patients might best be accomplished as it was a quarter century ago, by judicious use of rapidly-acting barbiturates, such as a parenteral dose of pentobarbital sodium, or one of the newer sedative drugs, such as diazepam. Normal persons find the side effects of antipsychotics to be highly disagreeable, and suffer from the side effects of treatment long after the precipitating situation is over. Even highly excited schizophrenics might best be treated with conventional sedatives along with an antipsychotic drug. The latter leads to potentiation of the sedation of the former as well as providing the desired specific antipsychotic action.

To use antipsychotic drugs for inducing sleep, rather than hypnotics, is completely unjustified in normal persons. They are not especially good hypnotics, and are generally more dangerous and more expensive than usual hypnotics. Often, one may wish to exploit the sleep-producing effects of these drugs in schizophrenics or some patients with disordered sleep associated with psychoses of old age, but hypnosis is never a primary indication. The use of antipsychotics in fractional doses for treating anxiety or depression will be discussed later on.

Rational Selection of Drugs

With the exceptions of mepazine and promazine, both of which are too weak in antipsychotic action to justify their hazards, the remaining phenothiazine derivatives have been repeatedly found to be equally efficacious when the responses of groups of patients have been compared. Still, individual patients respond differently to these drugs, doing poorly on some and better on others. The more sedative phenothiazines, such as chlorpromazine or thioridazine, were thought initially to be preferable for patients with agitation; less sedative drugs, such as trifluoperazine and perphenazine, being considered as drugs best for patients with symptoms of withdrawal and retardation. Such a differential action was based more on armchair reasoning than on experimental evidence.

A few systematic approaches to the problem have been attempted with uncertain results. Schizophrenics were divided into three types, "paranoid," "core," and "depressed," using pattern probability models based on presenting signs and symptoms. All three schizophrenic subtypes responded equally to perphenazine, but paranoid patients responded more favorably to acetophenazine. A later study by the same group failed to replicate such a difference, indicating rather that paranoid patients in general tended to respond somewhat better than the other types (104). Data from both VA study and National Institute of Mental Health Cooperative Study indicated that regression equations could be derived which might be expected to predict the most suitable drug (either chlorpromazine or fluphenazine) for patients with a given initial profile of symptoms. When tested against actual results, the interactions were significant. A later attempt to replicate this approach was unsuccessful (71). Schizophrenics were divided into four types, "core," "paranoid," "bizarre," and "depressive," and the actions of three phenothiazines were compared in each. Evidence was suggestive that chlorpromazine was the most efficacious for core, acetophenazine for bizarre and depressive, acetophenazine and chlorpromazine more effective than fluphenazine in paranoid, and fluphenazine most suitable for depressives. A later attempt by the principal members of the same group failed to replicate these findings of specificity of action of antipsychotic drugs (77). The general conclusion at the moment is that it is difficult to make a case for specific indications for antipsychotic drugs other than the original simplistic notion based on the sedative/antipsychotic ratio.

One is left, then, with a bewildering array of drugs from which to choose for an empirical trial in a given patient. Such a situation is analogous to the case of the numerous corticosteroids, antihistaminics, diuretics, and digitalis preparations which confront the clinician. The usual dictum has been to learn to use a few drugs well rather than all poorly. The differences between the proper and improper use of a drug will probably exceed any actual difference between drugs. One of the most rational ways to narrow the choice of antipsychotics would be to master one of each of the three types of phenothiazines, one of the two thioxanthenes, and a butyrophenone. With five drugs chosen on this basis, one should be able to exploit the full range of pharmacological differences between the various antipsychotics. Table 2-III shows one possible basis for such a choice of five drugs from three different chemical classes. Overriding all other considerations is the patient's past history of response to a drug, if that information is available.

The patient's past experience is quite a reliable guide. If he has done well previously on some drug, and especially if he has done less well on others, one would be foolhardy to change drugs or to reinstitute lapsed treatment with a different drug. To the objective response of the patient must also be added his subjective response. Unless a patient tolerates a drug well, he is not likely to maintain treatment faithfully. A patient who is made unbearably restless by a drug may much prefer no drug. On the other hand, some patients may prefer restlessness rather than impairment of their sexual capacity. The importance of various side effects to the patient should be a guide to choosing his specific treatment.

Doses

Few drugs have such great therapeutic margins and such a wide

Table 2-III

Rational Choice of Antipsychotic Drugs

Criteria: Example of chemical class
Different pharmacological profile

Types:
  1) Aliphatic phenothiazine – chlorpromazine
  2) Piperidine phenothiazine – thioridazine
  3) Piperazine phenothiazine – many
  4) Thioxanthene – thiothixene
  5) Butyrophenone – haloperidol

Majro Guide: Patient's prior response

range of therapeutic doses as these (Table 2-IV). Differences in daily doses of 20- to 30-fold have been recorded. Requirements of most patients fall within a narrower range, usually from 200 to 800 mg daily based on chlorpromazine doses. Occasional patients may do well with higher doses. One study indicates that doses of 2,000 mg daily may enhance improvement in some chronic schizophrenics under the age of 40 years who have been hospitalized less than 10 years (181). While no patient should be considered a drug failure without an intensive course of therapy,

Table 2-IV

Dosage Relationships Among Antipsychotic Drugs

Generic Names	Relative Potency	Total Daily Dose in Mgs	
		Outpatient Range	Hosp. Range
Phenothiazine Derivatives			
Aliphatic			
chlorpromazine	100	50-400	200-1600
triflupromazine	25	50-150	75-200
Piperidine			
thioridazine	100	50-400	200-800
mesoridazine	50	25-200	100-400
piperacetazine	10	10-40	20-160
Piperazine			
carphenazine	25	25-100	50-400
acetophenazine	20	40-60	60-80
prochlorperazine	15	15-60	30-150
thiopropazate	10	10-30	30-150
perphenazine	10	8-24	12-64
butaperazine	10	10-30	10-100
trifluoperazine	5	4-10	6-30
fluphenazine	2	1-3	2-20
Thioxanthene Derivatives			
chlorprothixene	100	30-60	75-600
thiothixene	4	6-15	10-60
Butyrophenones			
haloperidol	2	2-6	4-15

routine use of such massive doses may represent overtreatment for many. An idea, originally propounded in France, is gaining some credence elsewhere. Massive doses of fluphenazine (up to 1200 mg daily) may be given to refractory schizophrenics with relative impunity and with some degree of therapeutic success. The extrapyramidal syndromes so evident at lower doses of the drug disappear at these very high doses, for possible reasons mentioned earlier (195).

Assuming that the two novel pharmacological effects of antipsychotic drugs are linked, one might surmise that an inadequate dose of drug had been delivered in the absence either of an improved mental state or the appearance of an extrapyramidal reaction. A minimally effective dose of any antipsychotic drug should produce one or the other of these clinical outcomes. Neither outcome necessarily indicates that the best effective dose has been reached. Exploration of the upper limits of dose is based on other considerations.

Pharmaceutical Preparations

All antipsychotic drugs are prepared for administration in tablet or capsule forms of several strengths. Some are available in liquid preparations for patients who cannot or will not swallow tablets. Extended release tablets and capsules of several phenothiazines are offered to reduce the frequency of administration, but there is no convincing evidence that such oral preparations of highly cumulative drugs have any real virtues. In fact, they may have actual disadvantages in that plasma levels following some such preparations are often very low. Usually, absorption of drug is best from liquid concentrates, next best from coated tablets and least from capsuled pellets (107). Many of the agents are available in a form suitable for intramuscular administration. This route is the most reliable of all for making sure that adequate quantities of drug are made available. It should be remembered that drugs administered by this route are three to four times more potent than when given orally and doses should be adjusted on this basis.

A very long-acting injectable form of fluphenazine, the enanthate ester, is being used increasingly for maintenance therapy in outpatient treatment. A single injection needs to be repeated only every two to three weeks so that drug intake is assured. The principle involved in making this preparation is the esterification of a free alcohol group on the drug molecule with a medium chain-length fatty acid, effectively creating a new molecule. When deposited in tissues, endogenous esterases attack the bond, releasing the parent drug, but at a slow place. This principle may in theory be applied to any number of materials with a free alcohol group, having in the past been applied to preparations of various corticosteroids and sex hormones. Earlier fears that this preparation might release large amounts of drug unevenly have not been justified, although acute extrapyramidal reactions of the dystonic type may be encountered. The use of this preparation should generally be limited to outpatient treatment of patients previously well stabilized on oral doses. Some puzzling reports of suicides associated with the use of this preparation are explicable only if one assumes that it may have been given to suicidally depressed patients inadequately diagnosed. The present zeal for trying to manage all mentally disturbed patients outside the hospital should not blind one to the continuing importance of accurate clinical diagnosis.

The general practice has been to start medication with an oral dosage form, reserving parenteral doses for disturbed, excited or hyperactive patients. This practice developed because the intramuscular form of chlorpromazine was highly irritating. The advent of "low-dose" drugs has changed this situation, parenteral doses of these being comparatively well tolerated. One could now make a case for returning to the dosage schedule used in some of our earliest studies, starting all patients on intramuscular doses over a several day period and then following with an oral dosage form. One might then be far more certain of not under dosing the patient due to some vagary in his absorption or metabolism of the drug, or due to his covert refusal of the medication when given by mouth. A patient who shows less therapeutic effect than desired should not be switched immediately to another drug. A brief trial of intramuscular drug followed by oral doses with liquid concentrate, even without changing the previous ineffective doses, may entrance the clinical response.

Dosage Schedules

When starting treatment, divided doses are usually given. These minimize the initial impact of many of the unwanted pharmacological effects (sedation and adrenergic blocking activity) and allow better titration of dose. Unfortunately, this eminently sensible practice in initiating treatment is seldom changed, and patients may stay on divided doses for years.

As these drugs are intrinsically long acting, no pharmacokinetic basis for divided doses obtains. Once a patient reaches a satisfactory daily maintenance dose, it is feasible to reduce the frequency. Many clinicians aim for a single daily dose to be given just before retiring, and even when they use divided doses tend to give the major dose of the day at this time. Two advantages accrue. The patient sleeps when he should, not because he is oversedated during the day. Second, he is less likely to suffer disabling extrapyramidal symptoms if the major impact of the drug occurs while he is sleeping. For reasons still not clear, manifestations of Parkinson's disease are ameliorated by sleep.

The technique of reducing doses may vary. Some prefer to eliminate the morning dose first, consolidating it with one given later in the day and then progressively doing the same to noon and afternoon dose. If very large amounts of drug are required for maintenance treatment, one may still prefer to divide the total daily dose, giving perhaps one-third in the late afternoon and the remainder before bedtime. In most cases, however, the goal of a single daily maintenance dose can be attained.

Maintenance Treatment

The antipsychotic drugs may be discontinued after brief periods of treatment of acute brain syndromes, some manic episodes and some acute schizophrenic disturbances. Acute responses of patients newly treated with drugs are variable, ranging from days to weeks. Most clinicians would feel that failure of acute or newly admitted schizophrenics to improve after 6 to 8 weeks of adequate treatment with a drug would be reason to try another. Newly treated chronic patients might require 12 to 24 weeks of treatment before a change of medication would be warranted. Improvement tends to be more rapid earlier than later on, when therapeutic gains creep.

As a rule, schizophrenic patients are placed on maintenance doses which should be as low as suitable for retaining therapeutic gains. Dosage should be reduced gradually to avoid a sudden recrudescence of symptoms. The minimal dose at which the patient functions best is preferred to an arbitrarily-imposed maintenance dose such as one-third or one-fourth of the peak dose. Long-term uninterrupted medication (over 10 years) has proved feasible so that one should not feel impelled to discontinue the drug except in the presence of a side effect of overriding importance. Dosage should remain flexible to permit management of the inevitable periods of increased emotional difficulty. The importance of continued maintenance therapy has been demonstrated by a study in which discontinuation of drugs in patients already in partial remission was compared with continuation of full or partial maintenance doses. Over a 4-month period, 45 percent of patients who were discontinued showed unmistakable evidence of relapse, as compared with only 5 percent on full doses and 15 percent on partial doses of drugs (27). A similar relapse rate was found in 40 percent of patients discontinued from treatment for six months. The rate was higher in those who required doses in excess of 300 mg daily (182).

Apparently, many patients receive higher than necessary maintenance doses of drug. Still, it might be argued that 55 percent of patients remain in clinical remission after being off drug for a substantial period and that "drug holidays" might be in order. The difficulty is that, despite the most earnest attempts, patients who maintained improvement could not be distinguished from those who relapsed. Consequently, the most practical approach would be to consider indefinite uninterrupted treatment for most patients. The consequences of doing otherwise are quite evident; lapses in maintenance therapy with antipsychotic drugs are presently the most frequent cause of readmission to a mental hospital following discharge. On the other side of the coin, the value of phenothiazines in preventing psychiatric hospitalization seems to be well established (58). A recent study suggests that maintenance therapy has little value for "good prognosis" schizophrenics, or for those severely ill, but is of most value for the indeterminate group in between (137). Still, most clinicians would not want to make such an arbitrary assignment a priori.

Omission of weekend doses of medication would reduce the burden on hospital staff, either to dispense drugs to inpatients or to issue small amounts of medication for use during weekend passes. From a pharmacological point of view, omission of weekend doses is quite feasible. One might simply give the same amount of medication over a five-day period rather than over the entire week. We rejected using this practice at our hospital on psychological grounds. To send patients home on weekend passes, which are usually a prelude to discharge, without drugs, reinforces the erroneous idea that when they are discharged they no longer need medication.

Covert failure to ingest medication occurs in a small proportion of patients while in the hospital. The number not taking medication or reducing the dose increases rapidly in the first few months following return to the community, reaching as many as 40 percent. The patient should be cautioned to continue medication even though he feels well, and should be reassured about fears of becoming addicted. He should be cautioned about possible drowsiness and interference with skilled movements, and warned against the concomitant use of alcoholic beverages. The patient's family should have the same instruction. Information should be provided to the family physician and pharmacist. An uninterrupted supply of medication should be assured. The ever-increasing number of patients discharged from hospitals on antipsychotic drugs poses a special challenge to followup clinics. The principles in the use of antipsychotic drugs are summarized in Table 2-V.

COMBINATIONS OF ANTIPSYCHOTIC DRUGS

Whether we like it or not, and some of us don't, most psychiatric patients today are treated with combinations of psychotherapeutic drugs. In my hospital, the orders for a schizophrenic patient often reveal that he is simultaneously

Table 2-V

Summary of Principles of Use of Antipsychotic Drugs

I. Treat schizophrenia, not lesser symptoms.
  a. Agitation – use barbiturate, often with antipsychotic.
  b. Insomnia – use chloral hydrate, major antipsychotic dose at night.
II. Carefully select dosage form.
  Initial treatment may start with parenteral dosage form followed by oral maintenance doses; assures delivery of drug.
  If only oral doses used, and results not adequate, consider brief course of parenteral drug followed by oral liquid concentrates.
III. Tailor dose to patient's needs.
  Clinically, doses that are effective have varied over a wide range.
  Two clinical indicators of somewhat adequate dose
    a. amelioration of schizophrenia
    b. extrapyramidal syndromes
IV. Dosage schedules.
  Initially, all doses divided, but not necessarily equal throughout the day.
  Later, shift major burden of dose to evening hours, possibly only to a single bedtime dose.
V. Maintenance treatment
  Indefinite for many. May still be interrupted such as "weekends off" or "drug holidays."

receiving six drugs which act on the nervous system, sometimes in opposing, sometimes in reinforcing, ways. Here is a typical drug smorgasbord: (a) Two phenothiazine antipsychotics, based on a rationale to be discussed later; (b) a tricyclic antidepressant, usually based on the fact that the patient is withdrawn; (c) an anticholinergic anti-Parkinson drug, usually administered routinely prior to the onset of any extrapyramidal symptoms, and, at least in the present example, gratuitously; (d) a sedative, hypnotic or antianxiety drug to promote sleep; (e) a morning or daytime dose of a stimulant to permit the patient to carry out his daily activities. It seems little wonder that one frequently hears of patients who improve when some circumstance or other leads to the withdrawal of all psychotherapeutic drugs.

The rationale for combining psychotherapeutic drugs is based on several attractively logical hypotheses, each with rather little proof:

1. When drugs of the same type are given in fractional doses,

therapeutic effects are summed, but side effects are reduced due to lesser concentrations of single drugs or the cancellation of opposing effects. An analogy is made in this instance to the combination of three sulfonamides, in which antibacterial effects were summed, but the decreased urinary solubility of separate drugs at high concentrations was circumvented by lower concentrations of three single drugs.

2. Drugs with different mechanisms of action for controlling the same disorder may have complementary therapeutic effects. Such combinations are widely exploited in therapeutics: digitalis and diuretics in heart failure; diphenylhydantoin and phenobarbital for treating seizures; streptomycin and paraminosalycilic acid for treating tuberculosis; and so on.

3. Drugs have specific effects on various target symptoms, requiring more than one drug to treat all the symptoms a patient may present. As psychotherapeutic drugs are always used symptomatically in our present state of ignorance, this argument is more persuasive than in branches of medicine where the pathophysiological bases for disorders or diseases are better known.

These hypotheses, often employed to serve frankly commercial goals, have persuaded clinicians to use the melange of drugs so often seen today. Further, the old axiom that the more effective a disease or disorder can be changed, the fewer treatments needed, still applies to most of psychiatry. Despite the value of psychotherapeutic drugs, treatment of individual patients if often frustratingly difficult. The tendency to try to do one's best for a refractory psychiatric patient often leads to the accumulation of many treatments, including many drugs. If we had highly specific anti-psychotic, antidepressant or antianxiety drugs, combinations would be used less. Thus, the tendency to use combinations is a measure of the inadequacy of present drugs.

Combined Antipsychotic Drugs

The idea that two antipsychotic drugs might be better than one occurred to some of us quite early. It was all the more attractive in that the first two antipsychotic drugs represented different chemical structures with somewhat different pharmacological effects. Despite the favorable results then reported from combining reserpine and chlorpromazine, my own study indicated that patients treated with the combination were somewhat worse than those treated with chlorpromazine alone and that the prevalence of extrapyramidal syndromes, such as akathisia and Parkinson syndrome, was higher (96). This conclusion was apparently shared by others, for subsequently that combination has scarcely been used.

The combination of chlorpromazine and trifluoperazine was actively promoted sometime later by a pharmaceutical company which just happened to control both drugs. The proposed rationale was that combining the drugs would increase antipsychotic activity but that differences in side effects would reduce their intensity. Chlorpromazine was considered to be one of the more sedative antipsychotic drugs while trifluoperazine was considered to be less sedative. (The idea that trifluoperazine had a directly stimulating action was completely spurious, based on its greater propensity to cause akathisia.) The reverse situation held with extrapyramidal syndromes, as trifluoperazine was highly potent and chlorpromazine less potent in evoking these reactions. A controlled study of the addition of various drugs to maintenance programs of chlorpromazine in chronic withdrawn schizophrenics failed to bear this contention out (32). Adding trifluoperazine to an established maintenance dose of chlorpromazine neither increased therapeutic efficacy nor reduced side effects. Even the addition of more total drug to an established maintenance program did not augment therapeutic efficacy.

Another combination which has grown in popularity for a different reason is that of thioridazine and chlorpromazine. These two phenothiazines are considered to be the most sedative of the group and most suitable for the management of agitated psychotic patients. The maximum recommended daily dose of thioridazine is 800 mg, due to possible retinal pigmentation with high doses, but this level often fails to control severely disturbed patients. Consequently, chlorpromazine has been added in doses up to 1200 mg daily, making a substantial total dose of phenothiazines daily. This procedure is basically alright, but one can think of others which might control agitation equally well or better. Twenty years ago, faced with similar patients, one might have used parenteral doses of amobarbital sodium to control agitation effectively. Using the barbiturate alone would not ameliorate the psychosis, but the phenothiazine might. Using these two drugs in combination would avoid some of the risk of seizures or extrapyramidal reactions attendant to excessively large doses of phenothiazines.

The above examples illustrate the basic principle usually involved in combining antipsychotic drugs. One tends to use drugs from different chemical classes or the different subfamilies of phenothiazines. In the latter case, one representative from two of the three major subgroups, aliphatic, piperidine and piperazine, is usually chosen. Evidence thus far does not support the notion that such combinations are any better than adequate doses of a single drug. Although it is widely believed that the "high-dose" phenothiazines are especially good for managing disturbed patients and the "low-dose" for managing withdrawn or retarded patients, even these gross distinctions in the indications for the drugs are far from substantially proven.

Antipsychotic and Antianxiety Drugs

Two things became clear soon after the introduction of antipsychotic drugs: (a) They were not good hypnotics, and (b) they were poor antianxiety agents. Accordingly, it has become customary· to use drugs such as chloral hydrate, barbiturates, meprobamate or chlordiazepoxide in extemporaneous combinations with antipsychotic drugs when either of these two indications was present. The same general principles should hold in regard to the use of sedatives or hypnotics in the presence of antipsychotic drugs as when they are used alone: maximum doses are best given at night to exploit the hypnotic effects; doses need to be highly individual; the duration of a single course should be limited to brief periods.

Combinations of thioridazine with chlordiazepoxide have been studied in both chronic and newly admitted schizophrenic patients, the goal being to enhance antipsychotic effects. Chronic schizophrenics benefited equally from thioridazine 5 mg/kg daily or a combination of thioridazine 2.5 mg/kg and chlordiazepoxide 0.5 mg/kg daily, in each case more than from 1 mg/kg daily of chlordiazepoxide (95). The same antipsychotic effects were obtained from one-half the dose of thioridazine when it was combined with an acceptably small amount of chlordiazepoxide, suggesting the possibility that at least the dose of antipsychotic drug might be lowered by adding the antianxiety drug. Without any comparisons between both dose levels of thioridazine alone, such an extrapolation is a bit hazardous. This risk was further confirmed by a separate study in which a fixed dose of 30 mg of chlordiazepoxide was added to the optimal dose of thioridazine in newly admitted schizophrenic patients. The beneficial effects of the antipsychotic drug actually were slightly attenuated by the drug combination as compared with the same dose of thioridazine combined with a placebo (91). Approximately the same conclusions were reached by the same group from a separate study of a fluphenazine-chlordiazepoxide combination (92).

Combinations of antipsychotic and antianxiety agents would seem to offer no advantage over the use of the proper single drugs for each specific indication. If separate indications exist concurrently for both drugs, they may be useful to a limited degree in combination.

Anti-Parkinson Drugs

Anti-Parkinson drugs are most often used in combination with antipsychotics. Many clinicians use them routinely, even in the absence of any extrapyramidal symptoms. Such gratuitous use of anticholinergic drugs carries some hazards, as their effects may be additive with those of the antipsychotics or the more strongly anticholinergic tricyclic antidepressants. When the latter are used in combination with antipsychotics, no anti-Parkinson medication is really required. One would prefer to await the development of a clear indication for treatment with any drug. Practical considerations lead to some exceptions to this rule. If the patient is to be treated intensively with an initial course of parenteral medication or high doses of oral medication one may predict that extrapyramidal reactions will occur and prophylactic treatment may be warranted. Either when anti-Parkinson drugs are used to treat a drug-induced extrapyramidal syndrome or when their use is prophylactic, one can discontinue the drug after several weeks of treatment with no return of the extrapyramidal disorders (128, 163). The practice of routine use of these drugs indefinitely results in monumental over-use of these drugs.

Surveys of Combined Drugs

A recent systematic study suggested that combinations of drugs, at least as used in hospital practice, were no better than a single drug, and in some instances, worse. Five hundred patients, treated with a variety of combinations of two drugs, were divided randomly into three groups: one continued to receive the combination, one received a single drug and placebo, and the third received two placebos. Men actually did better on the single drug or placebo than on the combination; women did equally well on the single drug or combination, tending to relapse more quickly when placed on placebo (156). Such an approach is somewhat crude, but at the same time, keeps reasonably close to the usual clinical situation in which combinations are used.

Megavitamin Therapy

Although large doses of nicotinic acid and nicotinamide were initially used alone in treating schizophrenia, now they are usually combined with other antipsychotic drugs. The initial impetus for using these substances came from the "transmethylation hypothesis" of schizophrenia in which it was thought that an endogenous psychotogen was produced from normally occurring catecholamines through methylation of the catechol groups. These two materials were chosen as avid "methyl receptors," presumably blocking the pathogenic process. Over the years the claims and techniques for using these substances have changed frequently. They are no longer used alone; they are often used with large doses of other vitamins, most frequently ascorbic acid and pyridoxine, and the present claim is that they affect the long-term course better than antipsychotic drugs alone. The most recent report on this type of use of nicotinic acid led to rather equivocal conclusions (14). Actually, the findings of the study were rather negative, but because it is impossible in any single study to cover all the possible ways in which a drug may be active, the treatment could not be categorically dismissed. One has the feeling that many of the patients who are most benefitted from this treatment are those who might respond at times to other measures, such as psychotherapy or placebo. These are schizophrenics whose illness is usually clearly delineated in onset, often in reaction to some evident environmental stress, and whose premorbid adjustment was good. On the whole, large doses of nicotinic acid and niacinamide have been well tolerated, although they may aggravate peptic ulcer, gout, diabetes or pre-existing liver disease, and are best not used in such patients, if they are used at all (160).

CONCOMITANT NON-DRUG THERAPY

The antipsychotic drugs are the foundation for an effective total treatment program of psychosis. Few patients who have been hospitalized for any appreciable period as schizophrenics ever function in a completely "normal" way thereafter. Accordingly, realistic efforts must be made to help the patient so that he can live in the community despite his handicap. The teaching of some type of simple occupation may make it feasible for some patients to lead reasonably productive lives. As native intelligence may be high in many severe schizophrenics, goals such as limited vocational rehabilitation are not unrealistic. More and more, it appears that classical insight psychotherapy, whether given by individual psychotherapy or in groups, is useless in schizophrenia. New approaches using behavioral modification techniques are a recent vogue. It remains to be seen whether these approaches add anything to the effects of drug therapy. Following discharge, the same emphasis on real-life adjustment, just as might be appropriate in any other handicapped person, should be constantly provided.

Antipsychotic drugs have been used effectively and safely in conjunction with most other psychiatric therapies. The lack of improvement of patients treated with ineffective drugs or placebos cast doubt upon the efficacy of other therapies, although the evidence was inferential. A direct test in the case of group psychotherapy has been made, with little evidence to suggest that group psychotherapy is of much value in the total management of schizophrenics, or that it interacts with drug therapy to produce a greater effect than the latter alone (82). More recently, individual psychotherapy of chronic schizophrenics and its interaction with drug therapy has also been studied. Although both in combination reduced the florid symptoms of these patients, psychotherapy alone did little or nothing for the same patients (86). The hoariest therapies of all, occupational and industrial therapy, were also found to offer little or nothing not afforded by other therapies. It should be emphasized that these are mere beginnings in the evaluation of the various approaches to treating schizophrenics and one should not over generalize. Yet, one thing seems clear: Drugs do not prevent any benefits from other therapies, and vice versa.

When compared to other available therapies for schizophrenics, the importance of antipsychotic drugs seems difficult to deny (151). Yet one would be loath to deny the patient any possible treatment that might ameliorate his condition or make his adjustment to the real world (not the contrived world of the hospital or community health clinic) more successful. The true dimensions of the disability created by schizophrenia are shown in a study which indicated that while there was an undeniable beneficial short-term effect in patients who received antipsychotic drugs as compared with those treated prior to their advent, the change in natural history of the disorder which drugs brought about was not so great when patients were followed over a three-year period (187). Obviously, we cannot rest on our laurels.

SIDE EFFECTS AND COMPLICATIONS

Most side effects from these drugs are attributable to extensions of known pharmacological effects. A few are idiosyncratic or allergic in origin, and at least one, agranulocytosis, is due to direct toxicity. After so many years of clinical experience with these drugs, most important side effects are known. To be forewarned is in this case to be truly forearmed; one should always have a keen sense of anticipation for possible side effects.

Monitoring for side effects is best done by close clinical observation rather than by routine use of laboratory tests. The latter may be useful to establish baselines against which subsequent departures may be measured, and from time to time during the first several weeks of treatment these may be repeated. Excessive reliance on laboratory tests to detect complications is poor practice.

Behavioral Side Effects

Oversedation or impaired psychomotor functions are clearly due to extensions of the pharmacological effects of the drugs, often compounded by additive effects with other sedatives given concurrently. The most common adverse behavioral side effect is akathisia, or uncontrollable restlessness, one of the manifestations of the extrapyramidal syndrome. This symptom is often difficult to distinguish from restlessness associated with psychosis, but most patients recognize it as drug-related. Rather than being an indication for lower doses of drug, it may best be managed by the addition of some drug which will curb it. The combination of anticholinergic and sedative effects found in diphenhydramine makes it an eminently satisfactory treatment for this disorder.

Many psychotic patients are discharged from the hospital while taking quite large doses of antipsychotic drugs without any clear evidence of greater impairment than if the drugs were not given. During longterm treatment, the sedative effects are tolerated remarkably well. Curiously, the drugs are safe in two respects: It is virtually impossible to commit suicide with them as the sole agents, and clinical addiction is unknown. The psychologic disturbances secondary to drug effects which may occur in some patients with certain psychodynamic configurations, and which may even be of psychotic degree, are largely unexplored.

Neurological Side Effects

Extrapyramidal actions in the central nervous system and antipsychotic effects are closely associated, but it is not clear whether the latter are dependent upon the former. Drug-induced extrapyramidal reactions may be manifested in three ways: by a syndrome resembling naturally occurring paralysis agitans; by a syndrome of uncontrollable restlessness known as akathisia; and by various dystonic syndromes, chiefly one resembling spastic torticollis. Age and individual susceptibility seem to be the most important determining factors. Dystonic reactions are common in children and young adults, usually appearing soon after the drugs are started (101).

The Parkinson syndrome is managed by reduction of dosage, administration of anti-Parkinson agents, or both. Daily doses of some of the effective drugs are: procyclidine hydrochloride, 10 mg; trihexyphenidyl hydrochloride, 4-8 mg; benztropine methanesulfonate, 4mg; ethopropazine hydrochloride, 40-200 mg; biperiden, 2-6 mg. It is frequently possible, and always advisable, to reduce or discontinue the anti-Parkinson agent eventually. Sudden cessation of these potent substances should be avoided since withdrawal effects may result. There is no logical basis for the routine preventive use of anticholinergic drugs as (a) only a minority of patients develops extrapyramidal syndromes of any consequences; (b) the potential toxic effects of these drugs are considerable, including mental confusion, dry mouth, blurred vision, and occasionally paralysis of bladder or bowel; and (c) the expense of treatment is increased. Akathisia may be alleviated by reduction in dosage or concomitant administration of small doses of phenobarbital or diphenhydramine. The dystonic syndrome is relieved by the intravenous administration of caffeine sodium benzoate, 0.5 gm, or parenteral administration of an anti-Parkinson drug or barbiturate, repeated if necessary after a half hour. Administration of the phenothiazine derivative should be interrupted briefly, and an anti-Parkinson drug given when treatment is resumed. It is then preferable to employ a phenothiazine other than the one causing the dystonia.

Newly appearing seizures associated with electroencephalographic slowing, which is sometimes focal and paroxysmal, may cause concern unless it is remembered that these effects are common with antipsychotics. Other bizarre neurological syndromes have been described during treatment, but these as well as those already mentioned, appear to be completely reversible.

Late-appearing dyskinesias are increasingly recognized in patients under longterm treatment with antipsychotic drugs. These are most often manifested by repetitive, uncontrolled movements of the mouth and tongue, often with grimacing, masticatory or fly-catching movements. Choreoathetoid movements of the upper extremities, repetitive tapping of the feet, or shifting of weight from one foot to the other, and truncal movements with postural disturbance are also seen (46). On the basis of numerous clinical observations, these must be judged to be related to drug treatment, despite the fact that some of the mannerisms of schizophrenia may be confounded with these movements. Older patients, especially very chronically-ill women, tend to be at greater risk. The cumulative dose of antipsychotic drug received, the previous presence of the Parkinson syndrome, and perhaps brain damage based on concurrent senile, or arteriosclerotic, or alcoholic brain disease are also predisposing factors. At times the movements may be so severe as to interfere with the patient feeding himself. The syndrome has been described as being "irreversible," but some degree of reversibility has been noted over prolonged periods of time. Nonetheless, it is most disturbing that cell degeneration in the substantia nigra and gliosis in the midbrain and brain stem was seen in the majority of brains from 28 affected individuals (34).

The syndrome may be unmasked or aggravated by sudden discontinuation of antipsychotic drug and, paradoxically, it is improved either by increasing dose or substituting other anti-psychotic drugs such as thiopropazate, tetrabenazaine, or reserpine (213). The neurochemical mechanism is believed due to excessive sensitivity of dopaminergic motor neurons after long-term treatment. This sensitivity might come about from an increased synthesis and release of dopamine by the presynaptic neuron, due to feedback from the postsynaptic neuron whose receptor for dopamine has been blocked. Another possibility is that some membrane damage occurs to the presynaptic neuron so that the postsynaptic neuron is essentially denervated and characteristic "denervation supersensitivity" to the neurotransmitter ensues. Either of these two mechanisms would explain the fact that more of the causative drug makes matters better, and less makes matters momentarily worse. It would also explain the failure of anticholinergic drugs, such as the anti-Parkinson drugs, to be effective in this disorder.

Management of the syndrome poses a number of dilemmas. One is loath to take the path of steadily increasing doses, especially with the possibility of inducing structural brain damage. As noted earlier, many chronic schizophrenics probably receive much more drug than they need to attain whatever degree of remission they may have. Gradual reduction of doses to the lowest possible maintenance dose may be helpful in the long run. One might even consider temporary periods without drug, and in some patients who show comparatively little benefit from drug therapy, doing without drugs completely. Absence of a family history and of mental deterioration distinguish the syndrome from that of Huntington's chorea. One is tempted to speculate that this model of that disorder may be as rewarding as the drug-induced model of Parkinson's disease was for the latter affliction.

Allergic or Toxic Manifestations

Cholestatic jaundice, which was such a feared complication early in the use of antipsychotic drugs, has now all but disappeared. It was generally mild and self-limited. Most of the cases were associated with chlorpromazine, and possibly due to some impurities in the early manufacture of the drug.

Agranulocytosis is a directly toxic effect of phenothiazines on myeloid elements in the bone marrow. Although some depression of leucopoiesis may be seen in almost everyone treated with chlorpromazine, only rarely does it persist long enough to cause agranulocytosis (173). Generally, it is associated with the use of "high-dose" drugs, suggesting that the fewer molecules of a toxic material one gives, the less likely one will encounter this complication. Elderly, white women are most susceptible to this complication, especially if they have initially low leucocyte counts (diminished marrow reserve) or if they suffer from concurrent medical illnesses. The fatality rate for this complication remains rather high, although its frequency has been much reduced since the trend toward using "low-dose" drugs.

Both jaundice and agranulocytosis characteristically occur early in treatment, the former usually within the first four weeks, the latter usually within the first eight weeks. As both are initially manifested by fever, an accurate daily temperature record might be the best early warning device. Close laboratory surveillance, with routine leucocyte counts done weekly during the first twelve weeks of treatment, has detected a few asymptomatic cases of agranulocytosis, but the yield is very small. One might still wish to have on record a couple of baseline leucocyte counts as well as a battery of hepatic tests, so that future comparisons can be made if either of these complications is suspected later on. For the most part, laboratory tests are of greater medicolegal than clinical value.

Skin eruptions of all sorts have been associated with these drugs. They usually occur early and frequently are transitory. Photosensitivity phenomena of the phototoxic type are often observed with chlorpromazine (12). They may be reduced in frequency by the use of protective clothing and perhaps by the regular application of a protective spray. The usual remedies for sunburn will alleviate lesions that appear in the unprotected. Contact dermatitis in personnel may be prevented by avoiding direct contact with oral preparations, including the containers, and with the syringes and solutions used for parenteral administration. A desensitization routine may be useful if these precautions are ineffective.

Autonomic Nervous System Effects

Among the effects on the autonomic nervous system the acute hypotensive crises may be especially troublesome. They can occur when phenothiazines are given to old and debilitated patients or parenterally in large doses to patients of any age. Intravenous administration of phenothiazines for the treatment of acute alcoholism is a practice to be deplored; fatalities have occurred. The anticholinergic effects of phenothiazines are usually simply bothersome, but occasionally death has resulted from paralytic ileus, the infection of a paralyzed bladder, or a fulminating oral infection. Like other antiadrenergic drugs used for treatment of vascular hypertension thioridazine may inhibit ejaculation.

Hypotensive episodes may be avoided to some extent by having the patient lie down for a half hour or so after injection. Blood pressure should be measured before and after administration. Treatment of the rare, severe hypotensive episodes includes the usual postural placement for shock, oxygen, and 5 percent glucose in distilled water intravenously. Epinephrine is contraindicated; levarterenol may be given intravenously until blood pressure has stabilized, though occasionally patients have grown worse with its use. Blurring of vision can be managed by the concomitant administration of neostigmine bromide 10 to 15 mg per day, the use of physostigmine in 0.1 percent ophthalmic solution once or twice daily, or provision of reading glasses. Obviously, it makes no sense to use cholinergic drugs systematically when anticholinergic drugs for the management of extrapyramidal disturbances are also being used.

Metabolic and Endocrine Effects

Most metabolic or endocrine effects probably are related to neuroendocrine stimulation via the hypothalamus. The appearance of gynecomastia along with diminution of potency of libido may cause great concern, especially if the patient is not aware that it is a side reaction. Weight gain, often to a remarkable degree, is a frequent concomitant of treatment (126). It bears no direct relationship to clinical improvement in the psychosis, and may in part be a derivative of hospitalization. Although impaired glucose tolerance or the appearance of diabetes mellitus has been sporadically reported during treatment with chlorpromazine, one cannot be sure of a direct causal relationship. Large gains in weight in mature persons predisposed to diabetes could account for such reports, and weight gain is a very frequent concomitant of treatment.

Miscellaneous Complications

Disturbances in cardiac repolarization are frequently associated with therapeutic doses of thioridazine. These nonspecific T-wave abnormalities are believed by some to be benign, as they are usually rapidly reversible. Still, the rare instances of sudden, unexpected deaths due to ventricular arrhythmias in patients receiving this drug and other phenothiazines, may indicate a more serious import (136). While an abnormal electrocardiogram alone might not be cause for changing drugs, any patient with a history of cardiac arrhythmia or one reporting brief fainting spells (which might be associated with runs of ventricular tachycardia) during treatment might best be treated with low-dose drugs. It has even been proposed that phenothiazines and tricyclic antidepressants may produce a cardiomyopathy that is especially dangerous to those patients with other concurrent types of cardiac disease (4).

Pigmentary retinopathy is another complication limited to thioridazine and is the reason for the ceiling dose of 800 mg daily for this drug. It resembles retinitis pigmentosa in advanced stages and the loss of visual acuity is sometimes irreversible. Pigment deposits in the skin, and anterior structures of the eye (anterior lens, cornea) are attributable to chlorpromazine. These may develop quite rapidly when large doses of the drug are given (183). A number of possible mechanisms have been proposed to explain pigmentation from chlorpromazine, including increased tyrosine hydroxylase activity, increased secretion of melatonin and formation of an adduct between chlorpromazine and melanin.

TOXICITY

Overdoses, either by accident or design, have led to only a few fatalities when antipsychotic drugs were taken. These drugs may be directly lethal for children, where management of poisonings is more complicated anyway. The few fatalities in adults are due to other complicating circumstances (51).

Progressive impairment of consciousness is the rule, leading from drowsiness to coma. Initially, patients may become agitated or delirious with confusion and disorientation. Twitching, dystonic movements, and convulsions are other prominent neurological signs. Convulsions may be toxic, clonic, or startle seizures. Pupils are miotic and deep tendon reflexes decreased. EEG's show diffuse slowing and low voltage. Tachycardia and

marked hypotension are the principal cardiovascular manifestations, although an occasional patient may have a cardiac
arrhythmia. The strong alpha-adrenergic blocking action of
phenothiazines may make alleviation of hypotension difficult.
Hypothermia is the rule, initially due to disturbance of
temperature regulation; later, with increased activity, fever may
appear, although rarely true hyperpyrexia; the usual ranges of
temperature are between 31° and 40°C. Late respiratory failure,
often sudden, has been the distinguishing features in fatal cases;
vigilance must be careful and prolonged, so long as severe CNS
depression persists. Prolonged shock and cardiac arrest have also
been causes of death.

As most phenothiazines are readily water-soluble, removal by
gastric lavage is feasible; as they delay gastric motility, lavage may
be successful in removing considerable amounts of drug hours
after ingestion. Once absorbed, phenothiazines are tightly bound
to protein and become rapidly fixed in tissues. Experimental
attempts to hemodialyze ^{35}S-labelled CPZ indicated little transfer
across the cellophane membranes. Thus, it is unlikely that any
dialysis procedure will be useful in ridding the body of absorbed
drug; the same is very likely the case with exchange transfusions.

Convulsions are best treated by intravenous injections of
diazepam or sodium diphenylhydantoin. The possibility of
increasing central respiratory depression with further doses of a
central depressant drug should be balanced against the anticonvulsant effect, and only minimally-effective doses used. Acute
hypotension, not responsive to forced fluids, may require the use
of a pressor agent; norepinephrine is the logical drug for
treatment, being primarily an alpha-adrenergic stimulant; other
pressor agents which have been tried with success are intravenous
dextroamphetamine and phenylephrine. Warm blankets and heat
cradles may reverse the trend toward hypothermia, but if one
overshoots the mark, fever will ensue; the latter should not be
immediately ascribed to some infectious complication in the
absence of other evidence (106).

SUMMARY

The advent of drugs which ameliorate the course of

schizophrenia initiated a continuing revolutionary impact on psychiatric thinking and practice. Besides ameliorating schizophrenia, antipsychotic drugs had another novel pharmacological action, that of eliciting extrapyramidal motor reactions. From the two chemical classes of antipsychotics known in 1954, we now have nine which share these two novel effects. In addition, all antipsychotic drugs have many other pharmacological effects, some of which are medically useful, others which are unwanted. These drugs have been most successful for treating schizophrenia, but less so for other types of psychoses. Evidence of their efficacy in schizophrenics is overwhelming, but it is still not easy to predict the response of individual patients to individual drugs or to drug treatment. More than with most drugs, routine patterns of use make bad use; the doses and dosage schedules of these drugs should be highly flexible. Combination of antipsychotics with each other or other drugs has not improved their efficacy. In our present state of ignorance, we must employ all other "therapies" for schizophrenia in addition to drugs, for as good as drugs have been they are not good enough. Side effects of these drugs are not well-known and can be largely anticipated. Curiously, some side effects have provided useful models for the understanding of other disorders: Parkinson's disease; depression; and possibly Huntington's chorea. One last virtue: the drugs are remarkably safe in overdoses. Still, we have many new chemicals, but few new drugs. We must use experience derived from these drugs to understand better the chemical disorder of schizophrenia and devise more effective and precise treatments.

CHAPTER 3

ANTIMANIC DRUGS

The bizarre increase in psychomotor activity, grandiosity and emotional lability which characterize the manic state are dramatic and tragic symptoms. In its extreme guise, a manic attack is clearly recognizable as abnormal; many of those afflicted with the disorder can recognize its onset. Milder forms of mania, often called hypomania, are less easily recognized as abnormal. Individuals so afflicted are often valued for their initiative and energy, rising to high administrative positions in business or politics. Most are eventually undone by overstepping the bounds of reality. Curiously, society's tolerance of manic behavior seems to be far more than for a similar degree of depressive behavior.

Manic attacks may occur repetitively with relatively normal intervals between, or more commonly may occur in cycles alternating with depression, the so-called manic-depressive psychosis. Mania may often be part of the presenting picture of schizophrenia, and some confusion between manic-depressive psychosis and schizophrenia has long existed. Patients who have initially presented as being purely manic have eventually been diagnosed as schizophrenic. Recently the opposite sequence has been described.

In view of the frequent confusion between mania and schizophrenia, seven positive criteria for the diagnosis of mania have been suggested, based on observable behavior (146). These include accelerated behavior, object-related behavior, distractibility, flight of ideas, prominent or conspicuous emotions, history of previous episodes or mood swings, and positive family history of either a mood disorder or alcoholism. It should be remembered that the thinking of manic patients may seem to be "crazy" and that paranoid thoughts are also part of the picture of mania.

The severity of mania can be rather simply gauged using a

56

3-point scale for each of three typical symptoms: (1) flight of ideas (from absent to marked, requiring no stimulus); (2) affect (from normal to constantly elated); and (3) behavior (from quiet and cooperative to excited and aggressive. Such a rating provides a scale of severity from 0 to 6 (45).

UNIPOLAR AND BIPOLAR AFFECTIVE DISORDERS

The wild swings between mania and depression, so characteristic of the manic depressive psychosis, have generally been thought to represent the extremes of a continuum of behavior, the normal state lying somewhat in between. These disorders are considered to be bipolar, unlike those in which only a single affective disturbance occurs, such as pure depression. A differing concept of manic-depressive psychosis is that both of its aspects are progressive deviations from normal, depression preceding mania. This concept derived from the rapid passage of some patients from one phase to another, with no apparent normal interval. Most favor is generally given to the bipolar hypothesis.

The separation of depressive reactions into unipolar and bipolar types is of some theoretical importance. If these are indeed different in their pathogenesis, then the therapeutic benefits of lithium carbonate for bipolar depressions should not be expected to extend to the others. This question has some relevance in regard to the assertion that lithium carbonate can be used in treating recurrent depressions without mania or even simple depressive episodes.

PATHOGENETIC MECHANISMS

The peculiarly episodic nature of cyclic affective disorders has prompted inquiry into possible changes in electrolytes, steroid hormones or catecholamines to explain the rapid development of symptoms. As yet, no pathogenetic mechanism of manic disorders is known. Extracellular water tends to be low both in mania and depression, and plasma cortisol levels in manics tend to rise as episodes subside, contrary to what has been reported in depression. All these changes are slight and fall within the normal range of variation (41). The norepinephrine hypothesis has been postulated in reverse for mania; that is, an excess of norepinephrine rather than a deficiency occurs at central adrenergic synapses during manic attacks. Withdrawal from treatment with alphamethylparatyrosine, a specific inhibitor of tyrosine hydroxylase, has been associated with transient hypomanic states suggesting a rebound phenomenon following suppression of synthesis of norepinephrine (204). Conversely, alphamethyl-paratyrosine has been used to terminate manic attacks. In this instance, it could just as well be working through dopaminergic mechanisms as through noradrenergic systems. Levodopa may actually aggravate manic-depressive psychosis towards the manic side (81). The many conflicting aspects of the pathogenetic mechanisms of manic-depressive and other affective disorders have been well-summarized elsewhere (228).

VARIOUS TREATMENT OF MANIAS

Electroconvulsive therapy, which was formerly quite widely used in psychiatric treatment, was effective in manic as well as depressive phases of manic-depressive disorder. This lack of specificity of response somewhat favors the unipolar hypothesis. With the advent of psychotherapeutic drugs, the management of mania was effectively achieved with a number of antipsychotic drugs, including chlorpromazine, reserpine and haloperidol. As reserpine provided a pharmacological model for inducing depression, pharmacological evidence was more supportive of a bipolar concept of manic-depressive psychosis. Further evidence came from the clinical experience that some patients treated with antidepressant drugs tended to move toward a hypomanic phase. Besides the antipsychotic drugs, experimental treatment of mania has been reported to be successful with drugs that antagonize serotonin, such as cinnaserin and methysergide, or with those that block the synthesis of catecholamines, such as alphamethyl-paratyrosine (24). Treatments of mania directed at alteration of biogenic amines are by no means definitely established. Attempts to replicate the efficacy of methysergide for mania have more often led to the conclusion that it is not as effective a treatment as placebo (45).

Although lithium was introduced as a treatment for mania by Cade in Australia in 1949, it was quite slow to catch on as a popular therapy. The unfortunate experience with lithium chloride as a salt substitute for patients with congestive heart failure during the 1940's may have scared off physicians. The enormous impact of other psychotherapeutic drugs in far more frequent disorders may have tended to obscure the drug. It has even been averred that because lithium salts could not be patented the lack of commercial value of the compound led to its suppression, a rather unlikely hypothesis. Nonetheless, it was not until the 1960's that lithium treatment of mania came to be accepted in most parts of the world.

SPECIAL PROPERTIES OF LITHIUM

Lithium carbonate (the usual form in which the drug is given) is a somewhat unlikely candidate as a psychotherapeutic drug. Most of the latter have multiple pharmacological actions, and almost all can be characterized somewhere in the sedative-stimulant continuum. Lithium ion seems to be devoid of any specific sedative or stimulant effects, its presence in normal subjects being virtually undetectable. Neither does it have any other major pharmacological effects, such as adrenergic blocking actions or anticholinergic effects. Thus far, the only proven therapeutic value found for the drug has been in the affective disorders.

The measurement of plasma or urine concentrations of most psychotherapeutic drugs is somewhat difficult and hardly a clinical laboratory procedure. Such is not the case with lithium ion, the concentration of which can be simply, accurately and cheaply measured in almost any clinical laboratory. Evidence so far indicated a reasonable correlation between serum concentrations of the ion and both therapeutic results and toxic complications. Lithium treatment, therefore, lends itself to a much more accurate system for monitoring dose than any other psychotherapeutic drug (70).

Finally, lithium has been proposed as a "prophylactic" treatment for recurrent cycles of mania and depression. If lithium should be effective, in a truly prophylactic sense, it would be of enormous theoretical importance. We have no other instance in which a chemical treatment has been able to prevent one of the so-called "functional" psychoses.

INDICATIONS FOR LITHIUM CARBONATE

Manic-Depressive Psychosis — Manic Phase

After some years of clinical experience with the use of lithium in treating manic episodes, it was clear that it had some therapeutic value. The major question was not whether lithium was effective but whether it surpassed existing treatments. This question was examined in a large cooperative controlled trial of lithium carbonate compared with chlorpromazine. Lithium was less effective in treating highly-active manic patients than was chlorpromazine. The slow onset of its therapeutic effects resulted in many more drop-outs among those assigned to this treatment. On the other hand, chlorpromazine acted quickly and produced fewer severe toxic reactions. Mildly active manic patients reacted equally to both drugs, but lithium was preferred due to less side effects (184). Smaller controlled studies which had pitted lithium against chlorpromazine had usually failed to show any difference in efficacy. Most studies in which lithium had been compared against placebo had showed it to be more effective (219).

Manic-Depressive Psychosis — Maintenance Therapy

The success of lithium for managing acute manic attacks led some investigators to evaluate it as a maintenance therapy. Patients were generally selected from those who had a past history of recurrent manic-depressive episodes and the frequency of episodes subsequent to treatment was compared with that prior to maintenance therapy (6, 10). Relapse frequency was reduced during lithium treatment, not only in cyclic manic-depressives but also in cyclic depressions with no history of mania. A prospective study of the prophylactic value of lithium was undertaken in manic-depressives as well as patients with recurrent endogenous depression with no history of mania who had been treated successfully with lithium. Patients were paired within each diagnostic group and were switched to placebo or maintained on lithium. Results were similar in both groups given placebo, where slightly more than one-half relapsed within five months. Remarkably, no patient provided maintenance lithium treatment relapsed in either group (11).

The methodological problems in evaluating maintenance treatment using historical controls are considerable and may lead to some artefactual conclusions (20). The prospective study, unless it has some built-in source of bias, is less easily challenged. Already some confirmation has been provided in a study of 65 patients treated in 4 different clinics (42). The large-scale controlled study mentioned above has been extended to cover this aspect of the maintenance use of lithium, but its conclusions have not yet been announced. Meanwhile, most clinicians faced with the problem of recurrent cyclic manic-depressive attacks would be inclined to try maintenance lithium treatment in the absence of any potentially better treatment. Even if lithium should prove effective as maintenance therapy, one must wonder if true "prophylaxis" has been attained or whether one has merely afforded "suppressive" treatment.

Schizo-Affective Disorder — Excited

Schizo-affective disorders are characterized by a mixture of schizophrenic symptoms and altered affect, either in the form of depression or excitement. They are still somewhat ambiguous, being neither clearly schizophrenia nor a form of affective disturbance. Possibly, they are neither. The peculiar combination of clinical manifestations makes it often difficult initially to distinguish these disorders from psychotic depressions or from the manic phase of manic-depressive psychosis. In one study, of 43 patients initially selected for treatment with lithium on the basis of a diagnosis of mania, 10 ultimately proved to be schizo-affectives when the schizophrenic aspects of their symptoms became more apparent (237). Because these patients may represent a group which responds differently to lithium than true manics, the large scale cooperative study on lithium closely distinguished these patients from those with true manic-depressive disorders. A comparison of chlorpromazine and lithium in 83 patients so diagnosed resulted in somewhat similar conclusions as with the pure manics. Chlorpromazine was more effective in the highly active patients, while there was little difference between the treatments in the mildly active patients. Thus, the indication for lithium in this group of patients is somewhat less than for true manic-depressives, although this treatment may be quite adequate for the milder cases (186).

Acute Depressions

The general experience in controlled studies is that lithium is not an especially effective treatment for acute depressions. Many studies used a cross-over design, with all of its attendant difficulties. One which compared desipramine with lithium in endogenous depressions found no difference (155). Another which compared imipramine and lithium found in favor of the former drug (63). It seems highly unlikely that lithium would ever displace the tricyclic antidepressants as a treatment for endogenous depressions, but it would raise some interesting theoretical problems if it were found to be effective in these depressions as well as in mania.

Schizophrenia and Other Disorders

The available evidence indicates that lithium is a poor treatment for schizophrenia. Lithium actually seemed to aggravate patients with schizo-affective psychosis in one study where chlorpromazine treatment was effective (118). A similar superiority of chlorpromazine and a tendency towards aggravation with lithium was found in another study in newly admitted schizophrenics (210). Mixed reports of good results from lithium can be found for treatment of almost all known psychiatric disorders. This pattern holds for any new psychotherapeutic drug, but eventually a consensus develops which better delimits the indications.

PHARMACOLOGICAL CONSIDERATIONS

Possible Modes of Action

It is fair to say that we do not know the way in which lithium alleviates mania. Three avenues of inquiry into the action of lithium are directed at its effects on catecholamines, on body electrolytes and water, and on cortisol formation.

The effect of lithium on catecholamine metabolism may be somewhat the opposite of the tricyclics. The latter drugs slow the functioning of the neuronal membrane pump which moves catecholamines in and out of the cell, while lithium appears to speed it up. A preparation of synaptosomes from lithium-treated rats showed an increased uptake of norepinephrine (37). Supporting an increased uptake of catecholamines is the observation that lithium increases the rate of intraneuronal deamination of norepinephrine, as evidenced by an increased urinary excretion of vanilmandelic acid (VMA), a deaminated metabolite, and a decreased excretion of the metanephrines, undeaminated metabolites of norepinephrine. No change in 5-hydroxyindoleacetic acid, the major deaminated metabolite of serotonin, was found (93).

Lithium treatment causes an increased diuresis of sodium, potassium and water, but this is only transient (111). Manic patients often have a high tolerance for lithium and retain more of it than do normals, suggesting that it may displace sodium and potassium ions. These effects of lithium may not necessarily be related to its mode of action, although it remains to be seen whether the electrolyte and water abnormalities observed in affective disorders are causally related or are simply epiphenomena.

The secretory rate as well as the plasma concentration of cortisol was increased in patients with active psychopathology under treatment with lithium (177). Such a mechanism does not operate in normals or in patients in remission. Still, this does not establish that it is related to the therapeutic action of lithium.

The many pharmacological studies on lithium have been extensively reviewed elsewhere (52).

Kinetics and Elimination

A considerable amount of data about the absorption, distribution and elimination of lithium ion is available. To prevent toxicity, dosage must be maintained within a critical and narrow range. Lithium carbonate is absorbed within minutes following an oral dose and is virtually complete within 6 to 8 hours. Peak concentrations in serum occur within 1 to 2 hours after the oral dose. A two-phase half-life in serum suggests some redistribution to tissue compartments with accumulation over successive doses (28). After chronic treatment the half-life in serum is about 24 hours in the adult and somewhat longer in the elderly. It is estimated that serum concentrations of 0.5 to 1.5 mEq/L would be found after 600 mg doses given three times daily in acute mania and from 0.5 to 1.0 mEq/L during long-term treatment with 300 mg doses three times daily.

The ion is distributed in total body water, but later shifts intracellularly against a concentration gradient. Various tissues concentrate the drug to different degrees. There is no evidence of protein-binding. Passage into the brain is slow, but when a steady-state has been reached, the cerebrospinal fluid contains about 40 percent the serum lithium level (175).

Lithium appears in the urine within fifteen minutes of a dose, peak excretion occurring in 1 to 2 hours followed by a slow decline over the next 6 to 7 hours. About 50 to 75 percent of the dose may be excreted within a 24-hour period and eventually about 95 percent of administered lithium can be accounted for by urinary excretion. Clearance of lithium is about 0.2 that of creatinine with clearance rates ranging from 15 to 30 ml per min. About 80 percent of filtered lithium is reabsorbed, somewhat similar to the case of potassium ion. Ordinarily, the rate of excretion is independent of urine flow and dietary sodium, but with marked deficiency of sodium much greater amounts of lithium may be retained (accounting for the diastrous poisonings which occurred when lithium chloride was employed as a salt substitute in sodium-depleted patients being treated for congestive heart failure). Once lithium therapy is established, the clearance rate for an individual is quite constant (174). Determination of lithium clearance is a recommended procedure for establishing the proper maintanance dose during prolonged therapy.

Manic-depressives are alleged to retain more lithium following test doses than normals. In fact, it had been suggested that one might use the degree of lithium retention after a test dose as a predictor of the response of these patients to the drug. Recent evidence suggests that this simple predictive test does not have much validity (220). It seems rather more likely that the amount of lithium which gains access to cells may vary between patients and that perhaps one cannot rely solely on plasma concentrations as a guide to therapy.

Poisoning with lithium can be fatal, largely from pulmonary complications due to coma. No specific antidote works. Treatment is generally limited to supportive measures and attempts to hasten the removal of lithium through saline infusions, forced diuresis and alkalinization of the urine. Severe cases may be managed by peritoneal dialysis, which increases the clearance of lithium quite well (233).

LITHIUM IN MANIA

Concomitant Treatment

Lithium must reach a threshold level in tissues before becoming effective. The full effect on manic states is not generally reached for five to ten days. The antipsychotic agents and ECT can control attacks more rapidly, and are often concomitantly employed initially in severe episodes while the lithium stores are being established. Both the antipsychotics, with their sedative qualities and capacity to produce extrapyramidal disturbances, and ECT with its hazards, complexities of administration and after-effects such as amnesia have disadvantages not present with lithium carbonate. In addition, there are suggestions that the latter has a specificity that produces a true remission rather than the symptom containment or suppression imposed by the other methods of treatment.

Nonetheless, it would seem prudent also to use an antipsychotic drug in manics who are highly excited. The choice of antipsychotic might be any that the clinician prefers, although some might aver that haloperidol would be most likely to be effective. The drug might be used only until the initial symptoms are controlled, or until lithium serum levels have reached a therapeutic range. As is the usual case, the doses of antipsychotic to be used would depend upon the clinical response. Initial doses might be preferentially parenteral to assure the most rapid control of the patient.

It remains to be seen whether more aggressive treatment with lithium alone might suffice for such patients. One might be tempted simply to increase the doses or frequency of dosage early on to attain more rapidly serum concentrations in the therapeutic range. Still, this might not necessarily make for a more rapid response, as it may take some time for lithium to exchange with other ions within cells or in the extracellular fluid.

Dose, Dosage Schedule and Maintenance Therapy

As a rule, in treating acute mania, lithium carbonate (commonly prepared in 300 mg capsules) should be started with divided oral doses of 600 to 900 mg per day, rising to 1200 to 1800 mg on the next day, with adjustment thereafter in the range of 1500 to 2500 mg per day dependent upon the patient's course. This pattern of administration will usually produce the desired blood levels of 0.8 to 1.6 mEq/liter. Above the higher figure, side effects are more frequent; above 2.0 mEq/liter, more serious toxic manifestations are likely, so this becomes the upper limit. Since there is some evidence that individuals can tolerate two to three times more lithium when manic than when in remission, the physician might anticipate reduction of the therapeutic dose when the manic episode subsides (204).

After the acute phase has been controlled, and sometimes with outpatients in remission, a prophylactic dose may be established using a blood level of 0.8 to 1.2 mEq/liter as a guide. The daily dose may be as low as 300 mg but will usually be between 500 and 1500 mg per day. In the outpatient phase, the patient should be urged to take his medication faithfully, since relapses have occurred after years when medication was interrupted, and precisely as prescribed, since toxicity is just a few tenths of a mEq/liter away. An extra capsule or two when the patient feels it is advisable may prove just enough to bring on toxic symptoms.

The decision of whether or not to undertake maintenance therapy will be determined by the past course of the illness. If the attack of mania being treated is the patient's first, then one would prefer to terminate treatment after the attack has subsided. One might even wish to avoid maintenance therapy in patients who have only infrequent attacks. The general rule in attempting to evaluate "prophylactic" therapy has been to accept only those patients who have had two attacks of mania within a single year. It hardly seems advantageous to embark on longterm treatment if the attacks are less frequent. Efforts might better be spent in alerting the patient to the initial signs of a recurrence and providing for prompt treatment when it occurs. Curiously, some patients with minor degrees of mania prefer to be that way rather than accept maintenance therapy with lithium and a more "normal" state (179).

Monitoring Serum Lithium Concentrations

The importance of the blood level in following treatment with lithium warrants some specific suggestions. The emission flame photometer in the clinical laboratory can be equipped to do as adequate a job of measurement as it does for sodium and potassium. Measurements should be made on blood drawn eight to twelve hours after the last dose, since the guiding levels were so established. The rapid absorption of the drug means its peak level is reached two to four hours after ingestion, and that levels determined within less than eight hours will be relatively high. On the excretory side, the serum lithium level drops by about one half each day off medication, so that a low level may mean only a few missed doses, and an adequate level tells nothing about the way medication was taken prior to the preceding three or four days. During the treatment of the acute states, levels should be determined at least two, and preferably three, times per week. When the maintenance dose has been established, levels should be obtained at monthly intervals. Lithium has been given for several years now without the development of tolerance or of withdrawal symptoms upon discontinuation.

The usual serum lithium levels recommended for treatment have been somewhat modified by the experience obtained in the large-scale cooperative trial of lithium. The findings from this study suggested that 1.4 mEq/L should be the maximum therapeutic level during acute attacks and that levels under 0.9 mEq/L were likely to be ineffective even in mildly disturbed patients (185). While these may indeed be good guidelines, biological variability being what it is, I should guess that the wise clinician would not adhere to any laboratory test that was not consonant with his observations of the patient. The serum concentration may not always reflect the concentration at the site that the drug acts, and even with the best correlations between plasma concentrations of drugs and clinical effects notable exceptions do occur. Some general principles in the use of lithium ion are summarized in Table 3-I.

SIDE EFFECTS AND COMPLICATIONS

Before beginning lithium administration, the physician should perform a complete physical examination with special attention to

Table 3-I

Principles in Use of Lithium Ion

Indications
    a. Acute manic attack – established
    b. Recurrent mania and depressions – possible

Acute treatment
    a. Slow onset until therapeutic plasma concentrations of lithium have been established (0.9 to 1.4 meq/L)
    b. May require concomitant antipsychotic drugs early
    c. Divided doses
    d. Monitor plasma concentrations frequently

Subchronic and maintenance treatment
    a. Rarely requires other antipsychotic drugs
    b. Plasma concentrations about 50% of levels above
    c. Normal lithium renal clearance should be established
    d. Doses need not be divided
    e. Toxic symptoms appear over 1.6 meq/L concentrations

careful palpation of the thyroid gland. He should also obtain a total and differential leucocyte count, a complete urinalysis, a hemoglobin estimate, and clinical measurement of liver, thyroid and renal function.

The undesired effects of lithium can be placed into two categories related to dose and one that is not. Side effects can occur at any blood level, but are much more apt to appear at levels above 1.6 mEq/liter. They include gastrointestinal disturbances (nausea, vomiting, diarrhea and abdominal pain); muscle weakness; a sluggish, dazed feeling; thirst; polyuria; and a fine hand tremor. The first three seem related to peaks in the serum lithium, and tend to disappear in a few weeks as systemic adaptation occurs. The other symptoms may persist indefinitely, though they are reversible if the drug is stopped. All of the symptoms may be modified by spreading the medication over a full 24-hour period.

Lithium intoxication may appear when the blood level exceeds 2.0 mEq/liter. The central nervous system is the chief target. The initial symptoms, usually present several days before more serious ones appear, include drowsiness, muscle twitching or coarse tremors, and slurred speech. When unmodified administration of the drug has been continued, likely in the presence of impaired renal function, the initial toxic manifestations have been followed by coma, increased muscle tone, convulsions, and death from pulmonary infections. Treatment of this serious state is supportive and similar to that of barbiturate poisoning. Prevention requires thorough training of hospital staff, patient or family so that early manifestations of serious difficulties may lead promptly to further investigations.

Toxic situations require special attention in patients being considered for lithium treatment. The presence of renal or cardiovascular diseases may so interfere with excretion (a renal lithium clearance test may be helpful), or so alter electrolytes (as a result of low sodium intake) that the medication may present undue hazards. Advanced age also warrants special care, since the ability to excrete lithium declines with age and an effective dose therefore may be much less in the elderly than in the younger person. It is wise to increase the dose at a less rapid rate in searching for the opitmal level in the older patient.

Side effects not related to dose or plasma concentrations occur during chronic treatment. Diffuse thyroid enlargement may occur in patients on long-term treatment over a period of from five months to two years. The enlargement is usually moderate and associated with no change in thyroid function. Some patients have become hypothyroid or myxedematous. Thyroid function returns to normal if lithium is withdrawn. Administration of thyroid extract or other forms of thyroid hormones usually suffices to cause involution of the enlarged gland (76). A syndrome of nephrogenic diabetes insipidus may occur infrequently. Polyuria and polydipsia were noted early in the use of lithium treatment (206). These symptoms derive from a loss of renal concentrating ability which cannot be corrected by administration of vasopressin (188). More recently, leucocytosis has been observed during lithium therapy. Neutrophil counts are generally not excessively high, although some have exceeded 20,000 cells per cu ml. These changes are reversible and apparently innocuous (211). The use of lithium during pregnancy seems to be associated no more frequently with abnormalities in the offspring than the general experience. Congenital malformations were reported in two of 45 cases (5%), about the expected rate. As laboratory tests for teratogenicity of drugs are not especially predictive and are somewhat conflicting in regard to lithium, whenever possible pregnancy should be avoided during lithium treatment (78). Transient skin eruptions have been noted early in treatment, usually in the face, neck and intertriginous areas. The initial lesion is an acneiform papule which may ulcerate with coalescence. The lesion clearly is not related to toxic lithium concentrations in plasma (132).

RUBIDIUM – THE NEXT PSYCHOACTIVE ION?

Just as lithium can replace sodium in cells, rubidium can replace potassium. Reasoning that if mania, sodium and lithium were related, quite possibly depression, potassium and rubidium might also be, the pharmacological effects of the latter ion were studied. Rubidium proved to have a marked stimulatory effect on behavior of animals, and biochemical studies indicated that it increased the release of norepinephrine in the brain stem and that the released norepinephrine was metabolized to undeaminated metabolites, indicating an action at adrenergic receptors. Such an action is similar to the effects of antidepressant drugs, so a study of rubidium in depression was undertaken. Preliminary results are said to be highly encouraging (176). It would be rather astounding if such complicated behavioral patterns as mania and depression should yield to changes in the balance between those two major ions that determine the membrane potential of cells, sodium and potassium.

SUMMARY

Until a few years ago one scarcely thought of antimanic drugs as a separate category of psychotherapeutic drugs. The delayed recognition of the value of lithium salts in the treatment of manic states focussed attention on a specific treatment of these uncommon but bizarre disorders. Lithium is unique in several aspects: it is an ion, not a large molecule; it has no other pharmacological action than ameliorating affective states; it is easily measured in biological fluids; it may be the first chemical substance to be "prophylactic" against a "functional" psychiatric disorder. Its present indications are for manifestations of manic-depressive disorder, either acute manic attacks or cyclic mania and depression. Other indications, if they prove to be true, may seriously alter our conceptualizations of the whole group of affective disorders. Severe instances of mania may benefit from a combination of lithium with an antipsychotic drug. Serum concentrations (and perhaps even more, erythrocyte concentrations) of lithium ion provide an accurate basis for dosing and for maintenance treatment. Toxic signs are well recognized and not overly serious.

CHAPTER 4

ANTIDEPRESSANTS

THE disturbances of thinking and behavior of the schizophrenic or manic patient are beyond the experience of most of us. On the other hand feelings of depression and sadness are such common human experiences that most of us can easily identify with patients suffering from the manifold symptoms of depressive reactions. Still, it would be most unwise to confuse the symptom of depression, which most of us know, with the various syndromes of depression which, depending upon their severity, constitute depressive disorders. The latter have clear roots in both the patient's personality and life experiences, but not all persons subjected to similar stresses develop pathologic depression.

The symptoms of depression are manifold, and the initial complaint of the patients is quite often likely to be some common physical complaint rather than that of sadness, hopelessness or a feeling of failure (129). One of my colleagues said: "I can imagine a patient being anxious without being depressed, but it is difficult to imagine someone being depressed who is not also anxious." To be sure, anxiety, a feeling of dread or unknown concern about the future, as well as its objective component, tension, are virtually constant manifestations of depression. Somatic complaints, including loss of normal sleep rhythms, loss of appetite, and loss of sexual desire are frequent. Guilt is a feeling almost unique to depression. This constellation of symptoms, a depressed mood, anxiety and tension, bodily complaints and guilt constitute the basic depressive syndrome.

The frequency of clinically evident depressions varies, depending on the sources of data, the age groups surveyed, the geographical location under scrutiny, and perhaps even the time of year. Most estimates indicate an overall rate of about 3 per 1000 population (212). Very likely many depressions are missed until the most unfortunate outcome of all, suicide, supervenes.

Symptoms of depression may have a diurnal rhythm, being worse in the morning than later in the day. They may fluctuate widely over time. Depression tends to feed on itself, with melancholy breeding more of the same. A genetic predisposition is fairly well established and might have some relationship to currently fashionable theories for a biochemical substrate of depression.

ETIOLOGICAL CONSIDERATIONS

Since the clinical observation of depression evoked by reserpine, and the subsequent demonstration that reserpine depleted the brain stores of serotonin, norepinephrine and dopamine, biogenic amines in the brain have been linked to depressive disorders. The elegant "amine" hypothesis has not only proposed a biochemical substrate for depression but an explanation of the modes of action of some antidepressant drugs (43, 204). It should be recognized that the amine hypothesis is no more than that and that some compelling exceptions to it may occur. Still, it is one of the very few promising leads for establishing a biochemical substrate for an emotional illness and consequently has great appeal.

Besides involvement of either catecholamines or indoleamines in depression, other lines of inquiry have considered the hypothalamic-pituitary-adrenocortical system as a source of disturbed physiological function in depressions. Such a disturbance might affect biogenic amines, either in their rates of synthesis or their end-organ effects (50). On the other hand, decreased urinary excretion of cyclic adenosine monophosphate (AMP) in depressed patients, with a return to more normal levels with remission, raises the possibility of an end-organ disorder and perhaps a possible new explanation for the mechanism of action of antidepressant drugs (1).

Psychologically, most depressions involve a feeling of loss: of health; of wealth; of a loved one; of self-esteem; or of youthful vigor. One of the paradoxes of depression is that some patients who become depressed have all the outward trappings of success; their loss is their failure to meet self-imposed standards of excellence. The anger engendered by the loss may be directed inward, suicide being the most inwardly hostile action. Some psychological treatments are based on developing the outward expression of anger in depressed patients.

One might envision that depressive illness represents an interaction between environmental stress and some biochemical alteration in a specific individual. Persons deficient in central nervous system biogenic amines might be "depressive-prone." Given the proper environmental stresses, their coping mechanisms mediated by the central adrenergic pathways would prove to be inadequate and a depressive disorder would ensue. A normal person subjected to the same stresses might merely experience a transient feeling of the "blues" but be able to cope adequately. Just as with other emotional reactions related to life experience, depressive disorders may be treated with both drugs and with measures designed to alleviate emotional stress, either by "psychotherapy" in all its many guises, or by alterations of the patient's environment.

NOSOLOGY OF DEPRESSIONS

If one thing is certain, not all depressions are the same. Attempts to delineate differences between the clinical syndromes of depression have led to a ridiculous nomenclature. One hears of "primary" and "secondary" depressions. These must be akin to "endogenous" (which means "I haven't the foggiest notion of why the patient is depressed") and "reactive" (which means "I think I know why he is depressed") depressions. Another dichotomy, rather than being based on what may have caused the depression, is based on attendant behavior, being "neurotic" or "psychotic." Still another is based on attendant motor activity, such as "agitated" and "retarded." These dichotomies overlap: one could have a patient with a depression that is simultaneously "endogenous," "psychotic" and "retarded." In addition to these categories, we are still perplexed as to how to classify depressions associated with schizophrenic-like symptoms, such as schizo-affective disorders, or those associated with psychoses of old age. We are also uncertain about the relationship of manic-depressive psychosis, a fairly rare manifestation of affective disorder, to the whole range of depressive syndromes.

Of all the dichotomies in use, the endogenous-reactive has the most support and perhaps the most usefulness. Using a fairly simple depression rating scale, it was possible to show a bimodal distribution among a sample of depressed patients, with a more severe group, characterized as type "A," occurring in a previously stable personality, without any clear precipitating factors, and characterized by early wakening and being worse in the morning. The less severe type "B" depressions were opposite in these respects (200). A similar clinical justification for dichotomizing endogenous and reactive depressions (analogous to type "A" and "B," respectively) was cogently put forth some years before (125).

The advent of the digital computer, as well as systems for codifying symptoms, signs and demographic variables on patients with depressions, have led to new attempts at nosological classification. The most recent of these efforts yielded four distinct syndromes: (a) a relatively severe depression, often with delusional thinking, but with a good premorbid history (akin to the "psychotic" depression); (b) a moderately severe depression with high levels of anxiety, neurotic behavior and previous illnesses (akin to the "neurotic" depression); (c) one characterized chiefly by the presence of hostility in addition to other depressive symptoms; and (d) a mild depression occurring in young people with a mild background of personality disorder (170). To a remarkable extent, this classification verifies earlier separate efforts, in which depressions were characterized as "anxious," "hostile" or "retarded" (168) (see Fig. 4-1). The importance of making these separations of various depressive syndromes is that patients may respond differently to drugs depending upon which one is being treated.

The expected corollary to the notion that depressive syndromes may be clinically different would be that they might respond differently to drugs. Such seems to be the case. Although a limited number of drugs are termed "antidepressant," the wise clinician would treat his patient best by not limiting himself to these. Rather, he should approach the use of drugs in depressive reactions by examining the evidence for the efficacy of each in specific types of depressed patients.

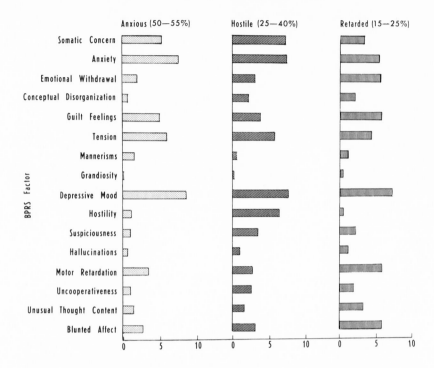

Figure 4-1. Three types of depressive profiles appearing in hospitalized patients with depression rated on the Brief Psychiatric Rating Scale. Relative frequency of each type shown at top.

CHEMICAL AND PHARMACOLOGICAL PROPERTIES OF ANTIDEPRESSANTS

Chemical Structures

Two new classes of chemical compounds, the tricyclic drugs and the monoamine oxidase (MAO) inhibitors, as well as the older sympathomimetic stimulants, may be considered as antidepressants. As will shortly become evident, other drug classes may also vie for this description, but these will be described elsewhere.

The dibenzazepine nucleus bears a great resemblance to the phenothiazine nucleus, although the spatial configuration may be more different than is apparent in a two-dimensional representation (Fig. 4-2). A group of dibenzocycloheptadiene derivatives,

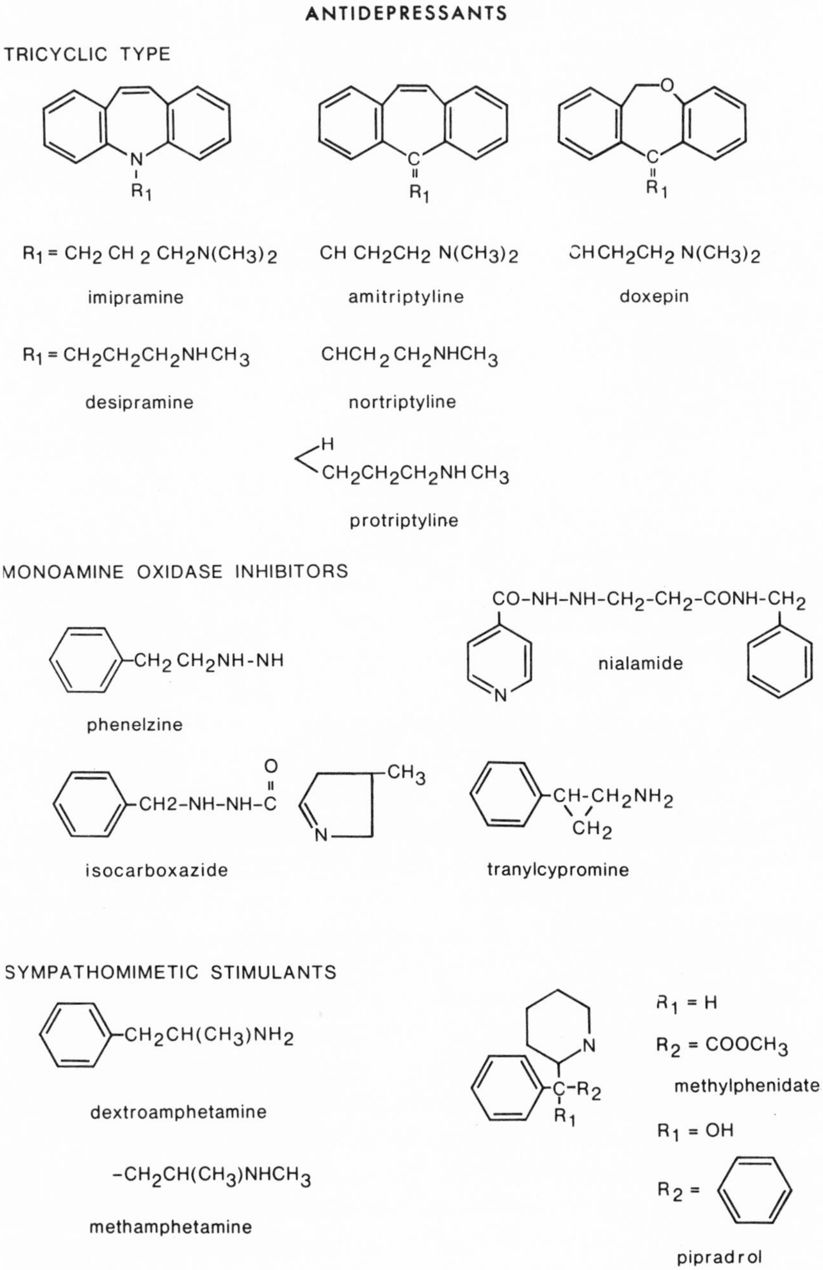

ANTIDEPRESSANTS

TRICYCLIC TYPE

R₁ = CH₂ CH₂ CH₂N(CH₃)₂ ... imipramine

$R_1 = CH_2 CH_2 CH_2N(CH_3)_2$

imipramine

$CH\,CH_2CH_2\,N(CH_3)_2$

amitriptyline

$CHCH_2CH_2\,N(CH_3)_2$

doxepin

$R_1 = CH_2CH_2CH_2NHCH_3$

desipramine

$CHCH_2\,CH_2NHCH_3$

nortriptyline

$\overset{H}{<}CH_2CH_2CH_2NH\,CH_3$

protriptyline

MONOAMINE OXIDASE INHIBITORS

$CO-NH-NH-CH_2-CH_2-CONH-CH_2$

nialamide

$-CH_2\,CH_2NH-NH$

phenelzine

$-CH2-NH-NH-\overset{O}{\overset{||}{C}}$ ... CH_3 ... N

isocarboxazide

$-CH-CH_2NH_2$ / CH_2

tranylcypromine

SYMPATHOMIMETIC STIMULANTS

$-CH_2CH(CH_3)NH_2$

dextroamphetamine

$-CH_2CH(CH_3)NHCH_3$

methamphetamine

$R_1 = H$

$R_2 = COOCH_3$

methylphenidate

$R_1 = OH$

$R_2 =$

pipradrol

$\overset{N}{\underset{R_1}{C}-R_2}$

Figure 4-2. Structural relationships between three chemical classes of antidepressants.

made by substituting a carbon atom for the nitrogen atom in the nucleus, and a dibenzoxepin derivative, made by further substituting an oxygen-atom in the ethylene bridge of the nucleus, have appeared. Imipramine would be the dibenzazepine homolog of the phenothiazine, promazine. Amitriptyline would be the dibenzocyclohepatadiene homolog of imipramine, and doxepin would be the dibenzoxepin homolog of amitriptyline.

Because of the confusing chemical names for such similar compounds, the simpler term, "tricyclic" is preferred when referring to these drugs. The discovery that the monodemethylated derivative of imipramine was a metabolic product of imipramine with apparent antidepressant activity led to a great interest in these derivatives, which are now almost as numerous as the dimethylated compounds (23). This situation seems to be different from that with phenothiazines, where monodemethylation markedly weakens all pharmacological actions.

The MAO inhibitors are of two chemical types, hydrazides and nonhydrazides. The first drug of the former type was iproniazid, a drug formerly employed for its antimycobacterial activity. A later member of the series was pheniprazine. Both have subsequently been removed from the market because of intolerable toxicity. As part of the toxicity was believed due to the formation of free hydrazine, later variants of this group tended toward structures which protected the hydrazide moiety, as in the case of isocarboxide and nialamide. Although many hydrazides can act as MAO inhibitors, the group has fortunately not proliferated. The nonhydrazide MAO inhibitor, tranylcypromine, bears a close chemical resemblance to dextroamphetamine, having a cyclopropyl, rather than an isopropyl side chain. This chemical difference markedly enhances its ability to inhibit monoamine oxidase as compared with dextroamphetamine, which possesses this action only weakly. Tranylcypromine retains some of the sympathomimetic actions of dextroamphetamine, however.

The older sympathomimetic stimulants, exemplified by dextroamphetamine, were phenylalkylamines. Newer members of this group, such as methylphenidate, retain a phenethylamine structure, but the nitrogen atom has become part of a piperidine group. Most sympathomimetic stimulants, regardless of the particular chemical class, share somewhat similar pharmacological properties (150). Although these drugs are often not considered to be antidepressants, and indeed under the circumstances of their abuse for social purposes are often derogated as drugs of little medical use, they act in a fashion quite similar to some of the antidepressants and may be useful for certain types of depressions.

Pharmacological Basis of Action

Soon after reserpine was used clinically as an antipsychotic and antihypertensive agent, it was noticed that some patients became depressed. The depressive reactions to the drug often were indistinguishable from spontaneously occurring depressions. Many reactions persisted after the drug was withdrawn, necessitating electroconvulsive therapy. Some drug-induced depressions led to suicide. These reactions suggested that the drug-induced depression could provide a model for naturally occurring depressions. The discovery that reserpine depleted stores of serotonin and norepinephrine in the central nervous system led to the proposal that naturally occurring depressions might be associated with decreased availability of norepinephrine or serotonin at their respective synapses in the central nervous system. This observation also focused attention on the possible physiologic function of these amines in the nervous system and provided a hypothesis to explain the actions of centrally acting drugs (178). Presumably, if depletion of amines is associated with sedation, an increase in brain amines should be associated with stimulation or euphoria.

Iproniazid produced central nervous system stimulation and euphoria in patients with tuberculosis. In addition to its anti-tuberculosis activity, it was found to be a potent inhibitor of monoamine oxidase, an enzyme largely responsible for the intraneuronal oxidation of amines in the nervous system. When evidence indicated that treatment with iproniazid increased the concentration of amines in the brain, the drug was proposed as an antidepressant (239). Early clinical experience was favorable, and a number of MAO inhibitors were introduced for the clinical treatment of depression.

The mechanism of action of amphetamines, which were known to be effective central nervous system stimulants, was reinvestigated to determine their effect on brain amines (26). Pretreatment of animals with reserpine, by depleting the neuronal content of norepinephrine, abolished the stimulating effects of amphetamine. Amphetamine may act indirectly by increasing the release of norpinephrine, or alternatively, may impede the neuron's re-uptake of released norepinephrine (8).

Imipramine, with a chemical structure and many pharmacologic actions similar to those of chlorpromazine, initially seemed to provide an exception to the rule. Its clinical antidepressant action was surprising, for it had been synthesized as a modified phenothiazine antipsychotic. The crucial difference in action between imipramine and chlorpromazine was that the former potentiated sympathetic responses whereas the latter blocked them (89). Imipramine and other related tricyclic compounds augment sympathetic responses by blocking the uptake of norepinephrine after its release from neurons.

The present model of the central noradrenergic synapse and the sites of action of these drugs are shown in Figure 4-3. When a nerve impulse or drug activates the sympathetic fiber, norepinephrine is released from storage granules located at the ends of the fiber near the synaptic cleft. After synaptic transmission, most of the norepinephrine is taken back into the neuron for further storage. The norepinephrine that is not reabsorbed is catabolized by the enzyme catechol-O-methyltransferase to produce normetanephrine, or other aminated metabolites. Both of these actions are rapid, setting a time limit on the process of synaptic transmission. Within the neuron, synthesis and degradation of norepinephrine are in a state of dynamic equilibrium, some norepinephrine constantly being catabolized by monoamine oxidase. The end products of this intraneuronal pathway are deaminated metabolites, primarily 3-methoxy-4-hydroxymandelic acid (vanilmandelic acid, VMA). Thus VMA is derived mainly from the endogenous turnover of catecholamines. On the other hand, only release of norepinephrine at the synapse results in the production of normetanephrine peripherally and 3-methoxy-4-hydroxyphenylglycol (MHPG) centrally. The excretion of these

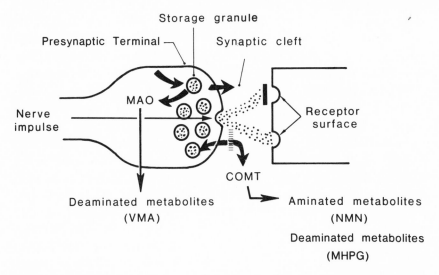

Figure 4-3. Model of central noradrenergic synapse. Constant intraneuronal synthesis, storage and catabolism (via monoamine oxidase, MAO) to deaminated metabolites (vanilmandelic acid, VMA). Neural transmission releases norepinephrine into synaptic cleft where postsynaptic receptor is activated. Transmission is limited by enzymatic catabolism of transmitter (via COMT, catechol-O-methyl-transferase) to aminated metabolites (NMN, normetanephrine) or deaminated, decarboxylated metabolites (MHPG, 3-methoxy, 4-hydroxyphenylglycol). Major limit of synaptic transmission is via specific amine pump which reabsorbs transmitter back into nerve ending; tricyclics and amphetamine block this pump (vertical cross-hatched lines. Monoamine oxidase inhibitors block enzyme, MAO, allowing for greater accumulation of transmitter in storage. Chlorpromazine and other antipsychotic drugs block postsynaptic receptor (vertical solid line).

metabolites is used as an index for turnover of released and physiologically active norepinephrine (9).

NOREPINEPHRINE HYPOTHESIS OF DEPRESSION

The norepinephrine hypothesis proposes that depressive reactions are associated with a diminished amount of physiologically available norepinephrine at the central adrenergic synapses (205). Antidepressants may rectify this deficiency through several possible mechanisms. On the other hand, drugs that provoke depression or control mania seem to reduce the amount of norepinephrine available at the synapse.

One can think of a number of ways in which the postulated deficiency of norepinephrine might arise: impaired synthesis; impaired release; increased metabolism, either through monoamine oxidase or catechol-O-methyl-transferase activity; or an increased activity of the amine pump mechanism by which released amines are returned to the neuron to terminate synaptic transmission. The implication of the theory is that depressions which occur on this basis are truly "endogenous," coming largely from within the individual and that they may be genetically determined. Increasing evidence suggests that "endogenous" depressions have a strong genetic component and are distinct from the manic-depressive disorders. The biochemical abnormality may simply put one at a greater risk of developing depression, the ultimate determinant being his life experience.

Is central adrenergic activity relevant to the clinical aspects of depression? In the 1940's, the Swiss neurophysiologist, Hess, postulated the presence of two separate centrencephalic systems analogous to the divisions of the peripheral autonomic nervous system. He labeled them "ergotropic" (sympathetic) and "trophotropic" (parasympathetic). The neuropharmacologist, Brodie, in the 1950's postulated that the former system used norepinephrine as its neurotransmitter and the latter used serotonin. In the 1960's, the Swedish school of histochemistry demonstrated that these two systems exist and that they do indeed have separate neurotransmitters. While we are still not certain what their functions are, it is quite likely that the physiological basis for what we might call "coping mechanisms" or "psychic energy" lies in the systems using the catecholamines as transmitters. Increasing evidence also suggests that most reward areas in the brain are noradrenergic. Two of the predominant clinical manifestations of depression are loss of ability to cope and loss of joy. Both these symptoms might be the expected consequence of decreased noradrenergic transmission.

The norepinephrine hypothesis of depression may be criticized on a number of counts. First, the data are indirect and relate to pharmacologic studies done in animals; in man, most study has involved urinary excretion of catecholamines and their metabolites, which may not accurately reflect events in the central nervous system. Until recently many of the products of amine metabolism which were measured in urine reflected more peripheral than central activity. The excretion of MHPG more closely reflects central nervous system activity but has only recently begun to be measured in depressions (147). Second, some investigators believe too much emphasis has been placed on norepinephrine, to the exclusion of other amines. Possibly, the dynamic balance between aminergic systems is of greater importance than the state of one. Third, some clinical exceptions to the rule have occurred; neither alphamethylparatyrosine nor parachlorphenylalanine has produced depression in man. The former, a specific inhibitor of tyrosine hydroxylase, should decrease the content of both norepinephrine and dopamine in the central nervous system. The latter inhibits the synthesis of 5-hydroxytryptamine (serotonin). Finally, the capricious effects of antidepressants in clinical situations contrast with their predictable behavior in the laboratory.

PHARMACOLOGICAL SCREENING
FOR ANTIDEPRESSANTS

The more or less fortuitous discovery of clinical antidepressant effects of drugs not expected to have them has once again created a circular trap. A battery of pharmacological tests has been devised from known drugs which may point to other drugs which are quite similar. The two main pharmacological screening tests for antidepressant drugs are (a) reversal of reserpine-induced sedation in dogs (one hesitates to use the term "depression" here, for the pharmacological and psychiatric meanings may be confused), and (b) enhancement of the vasopressor response to norepinephrine. Thy former test is positive with MAO inhibitors and tricyclics, but only to a lesser extent with sympathomimetic stimulants. The latter test is markedly positive with tricyclics with potent antidepressant action (but conspicuously weak with tricyclics such as doxepin with less clear-cut antidepressant as opposed to sedative action). It is much less positive with MAO inhibitors and sympathomimetics.

Although the EEG activity of antidepressants in animals has not been especially good as a predictor of antidepressant drugs, it has been averred to be successful in man. The resemblance of the EEG profile following acute doses intravenously in man of cyclazocine to that of the tricyclic antidepressants has led to its apparently successful clinical trial (65). As this was a generally unexpected effect of this drug, it remains to be seen whether the alleged antidepressant effect will be verified and whether it might be possible to verify this technique. Nonetheless, the general dissatisfaction with animal screening tests for antidepressants should impel investigators to look for new approaches.

METABOLISM AND KINETICS OF
TRICYCLIC ANTIDEPRESSANTS

The two principal pathways of metabolism of imipramine, the tricyclic antidepressant most studied, are demethylation and hydroxylation. Monodemethylation results in an active metabolite, desmethylimipramine (desipramine, DMI). Didemethylation inactivates the compound. Hydroxylation at the 2-position of the nucleus results in an inactive compound which is made water soluble by subsequent glucuronidation (Fig. 4-4). Thus, one may have any of these several possible combinations of metabolites, based on the three metabolic processes outlined (54).

The parent drug, as well as the major metabolite in plasma, DMI, is strongly bound to protein, with only about 10 percent being in the unbound form. Animal studies indicate that distribution is rapid, with relatively low plasma concentrations in comparison to those obtained in parenchymatous organs. Metabolism of the drug is intense, with about 50 percent being excreted through the bile and undergoing some enterohepatic circulation. Ultimately, two-thirds of the drug is excreted in the urine, mostly in the form of glucuronides; the other one-third is excreted through the intestine (18).

In patients being treated chronically with imipramine, the major material in plasma is DMI. Concentrations of imipramine and DMI are correlated with daily dose, ranging from 60 ng/ml of

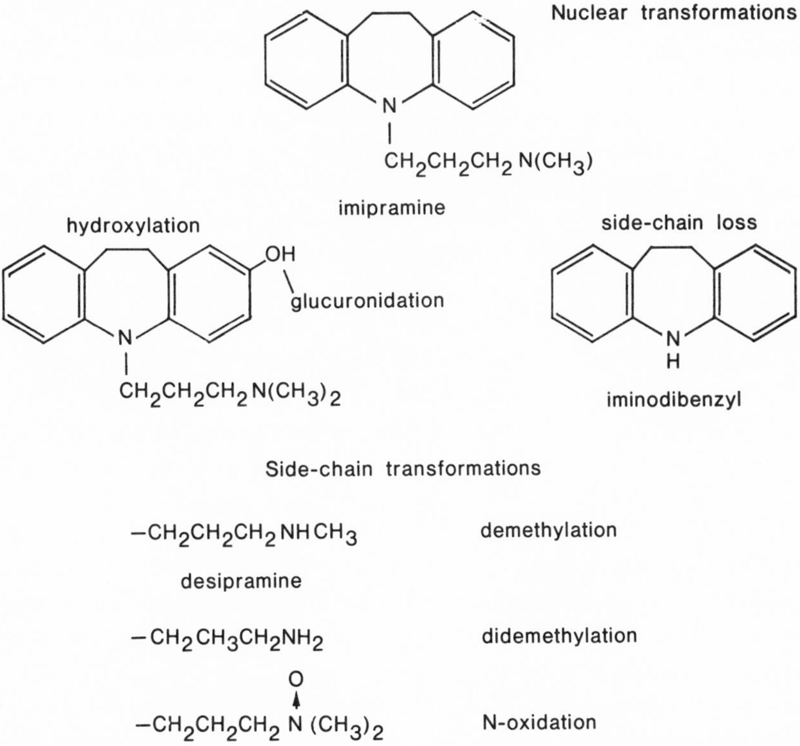

Nuclear transformations

imipramine

hydroxylation

glucuronidation

side-chain loss

iminodibenzyl

Side-chain transformations

$-CH_2CH_2CH_2NHCH_3$ demethylation

desipramine

$-CH_2CH_3CH_2NH_2$ didemethylation

$-CH_2CH_2CH_2\overset{\text{O}}{\overset{\uparrow}{N}}(CH_3)_2$ N-oxidation

Figure 4-4. Schema of metabolism of imipramine. Hydroxylation and side chain transformations are two major routes. Monodemethylation of sidechain produces active metabolite, desipramine.

imipramine and 150 ng/ml of DMI at doses of 50 mg daily, to 110 and 190 ng/ml, respectively at 150 mg daily doses. While ratios of imipramine to DMI vary somewhat between individuals, they are fairly constant within an individual. The same is true of the distribution of steady-state plasma concentrations of drug over a twenty-four hour period during which three divided doses are given. DMI appears as early as two hours after a dose of imipramine and tends to become the major material in plasma relatively soon. The variation in plasma concentrations of imipramine between various individuals given similar doses is from three- to seven-fold; for DMI, the variation is even greater, from three- to 13-fold. Chlorpromazine given concurrently increased the total plasma concentrations of imipramine and DMI, especially the latter (158).

The same wide variations in plasma concentrations between different individuals was found in patients given DMI. Steady-state levels varied over a thirty-fold range (only eight-fold if two extreme cases are omitted). The same was true for nortriptyline (NT), where a fourteen-fold variation was found. The levels of drug obtained were generally related to dose and the disappearance time from plasma related to level. Individual patients tended to handle different drugs of the same class in much the same fashion (215). The diversity between individuals as well as the constancy within individuals suggested that genetic influences play a powerful role in the metabolism of these drugs. Not too surprisingly, the handling of NT by identical twins was remarkably similar within pairs while showing a wide variation between them.

Correlations between clinical responses and plasma concentrations of tricyclic antidepressants suggest that there is an optimal range of plasma concentrations. In the case of 29 patients with endogenous depression treated with NT, the best responses were observed when the steady-state level was between 50 and 139 ng/ml. At lower or higher levels, responses were poorer. The suggestion was made that at high doses of drug a phenothiazine-like block of monoaminergic receptors might occur which would negate the presumed pharmacological action of importance (7). Another study which measured on the plasma concentrations of imipramine following treatment with this drug found that all patients responding to treatment had levels above 20 ng/ml (227). To a lesser extent, side effects and plasma concentrations are correlated.

The earlier observation of the effect of chlorpromazine in elevating plasma concentrations of imipramine and DMI has been followed by a number of studies on the influence of other drugs on the plasma concentrations of tricyclics and their metabolites. Initially, it was thought that chlorpromazine might compete with imipramine for binding sites and that the increased amount of unbound imipramine might allow for a greater fraction to be metabolized to DMI. Later studies suggested that the effect may be due to an inhibition of metabolism. Using ^{14}C-labeled NT, it was found that neuroleptic drugs increased the plasma concentrations of unchanged drug, decreased plasma concentrations of metabolites and decreased total urinary excretion (83). Aspirin, chloramphenicol or haloperidol administration in patients receiving NT caused a two- to three-fold increase of plasma concentrations of NT, evoking severe side effects. On the contrary, NT levels in patients receiving amitriptyline were greatly reduced during treatment with oral contraceptives along with a worsening of the clinical picture (196). Earlier, barbiturates had been averred to lower DMI concentrations, presumably because of their well-known propensity to induce hydroxylating enzymes. The converse, an increase in therapeutic effects from an inhibitor of hydroxylating enzymes, has also been reported. In this case the inhibitor was methylphenidate, which in doses of 20 mg daily augmented the plasma concentrations of imipramine and DMI (238). These same authors had reported a similar effect of methylphenidate on the metabolism of ethyl biscoumacetate and diphenylhydantoin, both of which are also principally hydroxylated, but others have failed to confirm these observations. If methylphenidate worked in the fashion proposed, it might represent a beneficial, rather than a detrimental, interaction between drugs, for it would also have a direct antidepressant action.

EFFICACY OF ANTIDEPRESSANT DRUGS

A few years ago, I wrote an editorial titled, "Antidepressants: A Somewhat Depressing Scene." The cause for my depression was the great difficulty in proving these drugs to be effective in controlled clinical trials. Recently, another investigator titled a paper, "Are Antidepressants Better than Placebo?" His answer was, "Yes, but barely" (148). Few areas of drug therapy are filled with more controversy and confusion, which is paradoxical, for as noted above, depression has the best established biological substrate of any of the psychiatric disorders, and of all psychotherapeutic drugs, antidepressants have the most logical explanation for their mechanism of action.

In retrospect, the two initial reports of studies with imipramine look very good indeed. The first report, by Kuhn in Switzerland, emphasized that "best responses were obtained in cases of endogenous depression showing the typical symptoms of mental and motor retardation" (131). The first report from North America, by Lehmann, also emphasized the particular value of imipramine in "endogenous depressions" (138). Much of the subsequent confusion in regard to establishing the efficacy of these drugs came about because the wise conclusions of these two excellent clinicians were not fully considered.

Few large-scale controlled studies of antidepressants have been accomplished and scarcely none recently. One of the first, a comparison between imipramine, isocarboxazide, a dextroam-phetamine-amobarbital combination, and placebo indicated that imipramine was slightly but significantly better than the other treatments. This study emphasized that all treatments showed considerable improvement over baseline, indicating the need to control for spontaneous remission, and that improvement would appear within three weeks in most patients who were going to respond to a drug (165). These findings have been repeatedly confirmed. A number of other large, well-controlled studies have yielded similar findings. Four treatments, imipramine, electrocon-vulsive therapy (ECT), phenelzine, and placebo, were given to 250 hospitalized depressed patients who were evaluated at four weeks and six months. The conclusions were that both imipramine and ECT increased recovery as compared with placebo and phenelzine (36). ECT was found to be more effective than imipramine, phenelzine, isocarboxazide, and placebo by a group with an acknowledged bias against ECT. As administration of ECT cannot be blind, the data overcame any possible negative bias (85). All treatments were found to produce substantial improvement as compared with baseline over a relatively brief period. A comparison of ECT and imipramine with placebo indicated that both were more effective but about equal to each other (236). The nonhydrazide MAO inhibitor, tranylcypromine, was compared with its analogue, dextroamphetamine, and found to be no more effective than the latter drug (167). The present tendency, therefore, is to consider the MAO inhibitors as antidepressants suitable only for refractory patients. As MAO inhibitors present real dangers due to inadvertent combination with other drugs or foods, the present cautious and restricted attitude toward their use seems well-founded.

One way to interpret the results of studies which show a small but definite superiority of tricyclics over placebo is to assume that they may be specifically effective for a small number of patients within the heterogeneous groups of depressed patients which are usually studied. Such an explanation was suggested by a study which compared imipramine, amitriptyline and a token dose of atropine as a control medication. Both amitriptyline and imipramine were somewhat superior to the atropine control, but the difference was significant only in regard to relief of a psychotic symptom, conceptual disorganization. Thus it appeared that these drugs might be particularly efficacious in patients with psychotic depressive reactions (100).

Because the pharmacological differences between the tricyclics and phenothiazines were less than their similarities, we decided a number of years ago to study systematically both types of drugs in patients with schizophrenic reactions and depressions. The phenothiazine, thioridazine, improved schizophrenics more than imipramine, although the differences were not as great as might have been expected. Surprisingly, depressed patients also improved slightly more on thioridazine than imipramine. These data were believed to show that at least one phenothiazine derivative was useful in depressions (166). Another smaller study, done at the same time, indicated that depressed patients treated with a combination of chlorpromazine and procyclidine (the latter to prevent extrapyramidal syndromes) or imipramine improved significantly more than those treated with a placebo. Both drugs were effective in retarded patients, while the phenothiazine was more immediately effective in agitated depressions (64). Applying computer techniques to analyze the presenting symptoms and signs of depressed patients, we were able to distinguish three depressive subtypes: anxious, hostile, and retarded. Using this categorization to reanalyze the data from the imipramine-thioridazine comparison, we found an unexpected drug-depressive subtype interaction (168). Imipramine was clearly the drug of choice for retarded depressions, while thioridazine was superior in anxious depressions. As the former comprised only about 15 percent of the sample and the latter over 50 percent, results from the total sample were skewed in favor of thioridazine.

A number of studies now suggest that tricyclic antidepressants may not be especially useful in mild anxious or neurotic depressions. In fact, neither imipramine nor chlorpromazine was better than placebo when compared in neurotic depressions, which suggests that these may be self-limited and respond nonspecifically (190). The same study confirmed that imipramine was better in depressions characterized as anergic or retarded, a finding that now seems to have general validity.

Intuitively, one cannot escape the feeling that a brief course of drug therapy might be beneficial for patients with a high level of anxiety associated with their depression. In neurotic depressed outpatients, best results were obtained from a combination of meprobamate and protriptyline only in those with low initial levels of anxiety (192). For most such patients, an effective antianxiety drug alone might be most helpful. Diazepam was as effective overall as acetophenazine in anxious depressions, being most suited for less severe and less complicated depressions (109). Characterizing clinical response to amitriptyline against four different depressive typologies, poorest responses to the drug were found in anxious depressions while the best response was found in psychotic depressions, as might be expected (171). Thus, the unthinking physician who routinely treats all depressed patients with a single antidepressant drug may be treating some of them quite poorly.

The growing consensus is that "retarded," "psychotic" or "endogenous" depressions (and they may simply be varying terms for the same syndrome) are best treated with tricyclic antidepressants. The value of these drugs in other depressive syndromes is more limited and may even be less than that of other drugs. In the most frequently occurring "anxious," "reactive" or "neurotic" depressions, experimental evidence suggests that antipsychotic drugs, such as acetophenazine, antianxiety drugs, such as diazepam, or even placebo may be as effective or more so than the tricyclics. Many of these patients might improve spontaneously in any case, so it is difficult to assign these drugs any more than an adjunctive role in treatment. As mentioned, the first report of the use of imipramine in depressions stressed that it was most beneficial in "endogenous" depressions. Now this clinical observation has been proved. The corollary of the efficacy of tricyclics in endogenous depressions is that the norepinephrine hypothesis may apply only to those kinds of depressive syndromes. As these are usually the most severe, and often the least clearly related to life experiences, the availability of effective drug treatment is an advantage. Still, the general term "antidepressants" embraces a broader array of drugs than is usually considered.

PRINCIPLES IN THE USE OF ANTIDEPRESSANTS

Indications for Drug Treatment

Drug treatment is not indicated for everyone who is depressed. Some patients require no specific treatment with drugs, while all probably require other treatments as well. Some years ago someone ventured the opinion that, on the balance, antidepressant drugs had done more harm than good, largely because they had caused many patients with serious depressions to be denied a prompt and effective treatment, ECT. The argument has some merit. On the other hand, many minor depressions, and some that look to be even more severe, improve spontaneously. A few years ago we tried an experimental design in one of our studies which we hoped would eliminate "placebo reactors" and increase our sensitivity in distinguishing between drugs. All depressed patients who entered the hospital and were candidates for the study were first placed on a week of placebo treatment. At the end of the week, the psychiatrist was then asked to make a decision as to whether the patient should be admitted to the study, based on the presence of residual signs of depression adequate to detect the effect of a subsequent effective drug treatment. We lost 50 percent of our potential sample, as that number of patients had shown a degree of spontaneous improvement which would have confounded the effects of future treatment (103). The tendency of depressed patients to improve spontaneously creates difficulties in the clinical evaluation of antidepressant drugs.

Many people suffer a "reactive" depression, precipitated by some life experience. The key word is "loss": loss of a loved one; loss of health; loss of job or money; loss of face; or even the paradox of the ostensibly successful individual who feels a sense of loss in not meeting the high standards he imposes upon himself. Some of these depressions require no more than a "benign neglect" or supportive psychotherapy. Older persons may become depressed following a surgical procedure (operations on the biliary tract are especially likely to precipitate depressions; recent evidence suggests that in obstructive jaundice the synthesis of catecholamines may be markedly impaired) or an attack of influenza. Rather than exposing them to the dangers of the potent tricyclic antidepressants, they might do better with a brief course of dextroamphetamine in small doses. While it is not fashionable to admit that stimulant drugs are medically useful, largely because of their misuse in a nonmedical context, clinical experience indicates some utility in milder depressions.

It is in depressions of moderate severity, regardless of whether or not the cause is known, that drug therapy may be most beneficial. Which drug to choose is best determined by the accompanying symptoms. If these are primarily bodily complaints, anxiety and tension, then treatment with antianxiety drugs may suffice, not only to relieve the attendant symptoms but also depression. Accompanying symptoms of severe anxiety or agitation, as in the "agitated" depression, may require an antipsychotic drug. In this regard, it is worth noting that in the study mentioned above, most of the 50 percent of patients not admitted to the controlled evaluation of antidepressants ultimately received some drug treatment for their symptoms. The most frequently used drugs were an antipsychotic in small doses followed by the two most popular antianxiety drugs. Apparently clinicians in practice have discovered empirically that not all depressions require "antidepressants."

The classical retarded or endogenous depression, as mentioned above, constitutes a clear indication for tricyclic antidepressants.

Should these fail, only then should a closely monitored trial with an MAO inhibitor, such as tranylcypromine, be considered. Should the depressive reaction be accompanied by obvious psychotic symptoms, making difficult the clinical distinction between a psychotic depression and a schizo-affective disorder with depression, then a combination of an antipsychotic and antidepressant drug may be used, such as perphenazine and amitriptyline. This combination is useful not because one drug adds more than the other for its specific indication, but rather than one drug doesn't much interfere with the other. One can have the best of both worlds, changing the ratio of drugs to meet emerging clinical symptoms which provide more clues to the correct diagnosis.

Severe depressions are one of the few psychiatric disorders with a fatality rate. Depression is often thought to represent hostility directed inward, against oneself. Self-destruction is the ultimate act of such hostility. To temporize with drug therapy and not to offer a treatment that has been proven to be rapidly effective in a high percentage of patients is a risk disaster. ECT is the primary treatment for any depression with a suicidal risk. Appropriate drug therapy can be used concurrently, there being some reason for believing that such combined treatment may both reduce the course of shock therapy required to attain a remission as well as sustain it longer. A schema based on the severity of depression as a basis for choice of treatment and drug is shown in Table 4-I.

Concomitant Non-Drug Treatments

It bears repeating that drugs should seldom be used alone. For

Table 4-I

Indications for Antidepressant Treatment

Mild reactive depression – "benign neglect"; supportive psychotherapy; brief course of dextroamphetamane
Moderate depression of known or unknown cause, with symptoms of:
    anxiety – chlordiazepoxide, diazepam, meprobamate
    severe anxiety or agitation – thioridazine, acetophenazine, thiothixene
    retardation – amitriptyline, other tricyclics; MAOI in failures only
    psychosis – amitriptyline-perphenazine combination
Severe depression with suicidal risk – *ECT* followed by appropriate drug

those depressions that are rooted in life experiences (and this may actually include all), "psychotherapy" or attempts to modify the patients environment should be offered. Extensive clinical experience shows that these maneuvers can be effective, either alone or when used with drugs. The case for the use of ECT has already been presented. Whether or not the contention mentioned earlier is true, that its benefits were being denied patients due to an excessive zeal for using drugs, it is safe to say that in many clinics this treatment is under-utilized. It is no longer a fearful or traumatic procedure.

Selection of Drugs

The first point in selecting drugs for depressed patients is to take one's blinders off. As pointed out before, one should be prepared to use a whole array of drugs, depending on the presenting depressive syndrome. Whenever possible, one might prefer to use an antianxiety drug over an antipsychotic drug in treating the syndrome of mixed anxiety and depression, and one of the benzodiazepines, such as diazepam, would be the first choice. A mixture of meprobamate and benactyzine, an anti-cholinergic drug, has been promoted for a long while, but evidence in support of its efficacy is meager. When an antipsychotic drug is to be used, doses should be kept within the tolerance of the patient.

The tricyclic drugs comprise a spectrum of sedative activity. Drugs such as amitriptyline and doxepin are highly sedative; imipramine is less so; the demethylated metabolites of amitriptyline and imipramine, nortriptyline and desipramine, are less sedative than the parent compounds; protriptyline is the only drug that has little apparent sedative action. It is still uncertain what contribution the sedative effects of these drugs have in relation to their efficacy in endogenous depressions. The more sedative tricyclics are increasingly promoted for use in mixed anxiety and depression. Nor is it clear what contribution towards the antidepressant action of these drugs is afforded by their anticholinergic effects. We often forget that most drugs have multiple pharmacological effects rather than the single one that we think is important.

The monoamine oxidase inhibitors act more like conventional stimulants. The most widely used drugs of this class, tranylcypromine and phenelzine, are chemically similar to the phenalkylamine stimulants, such as dextroamphetamine, but are much more potent as inhibitors of monoamine oxidase. These drugs, both because of their poor showing in controlled clinical trials as well as their many potentially hazardous side effects, are recommended only as drugs of last resort, for patients who continue to show severe endogenous depressive symptoms following an adequate trial of one or more tricyclic drugs. Their use should be restricted to patients who are hospitalized or who can be closely supervised medically.

An additional reason for hesitating to select a single mechanism of action for antidepressants is exemplified by dextro-amphetamine. From what is known of its pharmacological effects, it should rank among the more effective antidepressant drugs. Yet it was not a popular or highly-regarded antidepressant prior to the advent of the newer ones, and since then it is used even less. One would be loath to recommend this drug for patients with endogenous depressions, yet for many with milder depressions its euphoriant effects are beneficial. It may be a gross oversimplification, but a drug which produces true euphoria (by whatever means this may be achieved) may have some potential as an antidepressant.

Doses and Dosage Schedules

Ideally, one would prefer to monitor doses of tricyclics on the basis of plasma concentrations of the drug as correlations with clinical effects are reasonably good. The techniques of measurement of plasma levels are not yet simple enough to become a routine clinical criteria for determining an adequate dose. These criteria are either amelioration of the depression, the desired therapeutic end-point, or development of intolerable anticholinergic or sedative effects, the undesired end-points. Many depressed patients best treated with tricyclic antidepressants are in the middle or later years of life, when the peripheral and central anticholinergic effects may be a real problem. In their mildest guise, they may be only dryness of the mouth or blurring of vision. More severe manifestations may be urinary retention, paralytic ileus or toxic delirium. The latter is especially a hazard in the elderly. Still, the basic principle in arriving at a proper dose is to increase it until either the desired or unbearable undesired pharmacological effects are attained.

The usual pattern of dosage has been to begin with small, divided doses, such as 25 mg of amitriptyline three times daily. Dividing doses initially lessens the impact of the side effects, and increases flexibility in determining the optimal dose. This small amount of drug may be adequate for many patients, although the wide variability between patients in the plasma concentrations of drug attained requires one to vary doses over a range of six- or eight-fold. Incremental doses can be added daily or every other day, depending upon the urgency of the clinical situation. Many clinicians prefer to add 25 mg increments to the night-time dose of drug, rather than burden the patient with excessive day-time doses. For patients who are especially sensitive to the sedative effects of tricyclics, the major portion of the dose should always be given at bedtime. A single night-time dose during maintenance therapy, just as with the phenothiazines, may be used with tricyclics. Few patients require a total daily dose above 300 mg. (Usual daily doses of all antidepressants are shown in Table 4-II.)

It is often averred that tricyclic antidepressants take a long time to work, which may be true if doses are conservative and increments infrequent. With close attention to regulating doses, steady-state concentrations in the therapeutic ranges should be reached fairly quickly. One should see some benefits, if they are to occur at all, within a week or two. Should none be apparent by three weeks, assuming that one has scrupulously attempted to find the proper dose, one should seriously consider using another drug or another treatment. Among depressed patients, unlike schizophrenic, morbidity is an important consideration. One should strive to reduce the time the patient is disabled, as many depressed patients have responsibilities and must return quickly to their jobs, their businesses, their professions or their families. The demethylated metabolites, such as desipramine or nortriptyline, are said to

Table 4-II

Dosage Guide for Antidepressants

Generic Names	Total Daily Dosage in Mgs (Divided into 2-4 Doses)	
	Outpatient Range	*Hospital Range*
Tricyclic Derivatives		
amitriptyline	50-150	75-300
desipramine	75-150	75-300
imipramine	50-150	75-300
nortriptyline	20-100	40-100
protriptyline	10-40	15-60
Hydrazide MAO Inhibitors		
isocarboxazid	10-30	10-50
nialamide	25-75	100-450
phenelzine	15-30	15-75
Non-Hydrazide MAO Inhibitors		
tranylcypromine	20-30	20-30
Stimulants		
dextroamphetamine	5-15	10-30
methamphetamine	2.5-10	10-20
methylphenidate	10-30	20-60
piparadrol®	2-4	4-10

hasten clinical response, presumably by circumventing the need for these metabolites to be formed from their parent compounds. As this change occurs within the body in a few hours, the reasoning behind this assertion seems quite dubious. Clinical experience with the demethylated compounds suggests that they are not superior to the parent drugs, if indeed they are not less effective (55). Another way by which therapeutic effects might be attained more rapidly is through intramuscular injection of the drugs, as this dosage form is available for most of them. Although some clinical reports state that response from this mode of administration is faster than from oral doses, they are generally without controls.

The principle of dosage with MAO inhibitors is quite different. One uses a large loading dose right off and then seeks to find the optimal smaller dose to attain maximum therapeutic effects. As these drugs are intrinsically very long-acting due to their irreversible inhibition of the enzyme, single daily doses given in the morning should suffice.

MAO inhibitors produce their clinical effects presumably to the degree that monoamine oxidase inhibition is attained. Some commonly used dosage schedules may fail to inhibit MAO sufficiently. A clinical criterion which might be used to assay the degree of MAO inhibition is evidence of sympathetic inhibition, such as orthostatic hypotension, slowed heart rate, increased bowel sounds or abnormal responses to the Valsalva maneuver or the cold pressor test. Chemical evidence of MAO inhibition would be manifested by increased urinary excretion of tyramine or tryptamine, neither of which would be metabolized when MAO is inhibited. As very few clinical studies have used such controls to monitor dosage, it may be that these drugs are not as ineffective as they seem. On the other hand, the frequent complications from peripheral MAO inhibition would seem to indicate that not all dosage schedules are inadequate.

When sympathetic stimulants are used for treating depression, a single morning dose may suffice. These drugs are fairly long-acting, so that doses later in the day may interfere with sleep. One generally wants to start out with the smallest possible doses to attain benefit, possibly no more than 5 mg of dextroamphetamine. Any side effects of weight loss, unless this is desired as well, or insomnia are indications for stopping treatment or reducing the dose. Treatment might be given in a brief course of seven to ten days, interrupted by at least equivalent periods if it must be continued longer.

Maintenance Treatment

Assuming that one attains a satisfactory degree of remission from drug therapy, how long should it be continued? The best guide would seem to be the patient's past history of depression. If the attack of depression was mild, quick to respond, and the first one requiring treatment, one might be tempted to taper off treatment within a week or two after remission was attained. During this period, one should be especially alert to any signs of relapse, which might then require a slower pace of discontinuing treatment. On the other hand, if the attack of depression was one of a series which were becoming more frequent, more severe, and more refractory to treatment, one might consider maintenance therapy for months or even years. Many cases have been documented in which patients have been maintained free of depression on very small doses (usually given once daily at night) of tricyclic antidepressants, but who experience a rapid recrudescence of symptoms when attempts are made to discontinue the drug. The natural history of a disorder is the best guide to prognosis as well as choice of treatment. Some principles in the use of antidepressant drugs are summarized in Table 4-III.

Table 4-III

Principles in Use of Antidepressants

I. Do not neglect other therapies
   a. ECT may save a life in a severe suicidal depression
   b. "Psychotherapy" (of many different types) may be useful
   c. Environmental alteration sometimes helpful
II. Be aware of possibly limiting pharmacological actions
   a. Tricyclics have strong anticholinergic effects which may limit dose; also may be sedative for some individuals
   b. MAO inhibitors – numerous interactions
III. Choice of drug
   a. Based on depressive syndrome
   b. Past experience always the best guide
IV. Doses
   a. No set dose. Wide variations in plasma concentrations among individuals on same dose
   b. Dose to attain therapeutic benefit or limited by side effects
V. Dosage
   a. Small initially divided doses provide rapid titration and avoid intolerance
   b. Later, doses may be less frequent, or even once daily
   c. Should see some effect in 2 to 3 weeks; if not, consider alternatives
VI. Maintenance treatment
   a. Past history of depressive episodes is best guide
   b. Many patients require very long maintenance but frequently at rather small doses.

COMBINATIONS OF DRUGS

Combinations of Antidepressants

Theoretically, combination of various antidepressants makes sense (201). The three major classes of antidepressants (tricyclics, monoamine oxidase (MAO) inhibitors and sympathomimetic stimulants) represent different types of chemical structures. Although each leads to the same pharmacological end-point, an increased concentration of neurotransmitters at central aminergic synapses, they reach this goal by different mechanisms. Thus, they offer an ideal situation for combining drugs with different chemical structures and mechanisms of action. The fact that they rarely are combined may in part be due to over-emphasis of the dangers of such combination, as well as a failure to increase therapeutic efficacy.

Although three types of combination of antidepressants are possible (tricyclics with MAO inhibitors or sympathomimetics, and the latter two with themselves), only the former combinations have elicited any enthusiasm. Combinations of imipramine and phenelzine, for instance, have been employed with apparent success, but careful monitoring of dosage and patients is required; the doses of each drug must be lower than if they were used alone. Consequently, it is questionable whether any therapeutic gain can be achieved. Inadvertent, poorly-controlled combinations of these drugs have led to a syndrome of central sympathetic overactivity manifested by disturbances of consciousness, seizures and death, emphasizing the limitations of pushing these pharmacological effects.

In a sense, a combination of MAO inhibition and sympatho-mimetic stimulation was present in a single drug, tranycypromine. This drug is a much more potent MAO inhibitor than its close chemical relative, dextroamphetamine, but retained the latter's sympathomimetic action. Some cases of acute hypertensive episodes have resulted from using tranylcypromine alone, but many more were caused by the unwitting combination of this or other MAO inhibitors with sympathomimetics, such as tyramine, found in a variety of foods. The serious interactions from such combinations have been well documented and have led to the demise of MAO inhibitors as an important class of antidepressant drugs (214).

Combinations of two tricyclic antidepressants would not seem to be rational, as most have the same mechanism of action. The monodemethylated analogs of imipramine and amitriptyline, desipramine and nortriptyline are said to be less sedative than the parent compounds, but equally effective as antidepressants. An uncontrolled trial of the sequential combination of nortriptyline and amitriptyline seemed to show efficacy of the combination, but no more than might have been expected from a single drug (87). A slightly different analog, protriptyline, seems to be stimulating rather than sedating. Combining protriptyline with a sedative tricyclic, such as amitriptyline, might balance the sedative-stimulant effects while summing the antidepressive action. One uncontrolled trial of this combination has reported favorable results, but again, the lack of control allows no conclusion that the combination has increased efficacy (240).

Antidepressant and Antianxiety Agents

Long before the emergence of modern clinical psychopharmacology in the 1950's, a combination of amobarbital sodium and dextroamphetamine was promoted as a "mood-stabilizer." This hoary preparation still retains a remarkable popularity. As each component drug has antagonistic pharmacological actions to the other, the combination might be thought of as a pharmacologically-active placebo. In at least one controlled trial in which it was tested in depressive reactions, its effects paralleled those of the placebo to a remarkable degree (165). Still, others have proposed, primarily on the basis of animal experimentation, that the combination results in a novel pharmacological effect not attributable to the action of either drug alone.

While it may be possible to be anxious without being depressed, the converse is seldom true. Consequently, the clinical popularity of combinations of drugs which cover both ends of the sedative-stimulant continuum may be easily explained. At the present time, sedation must be equated with antianxiety affects, simply because no antianxiety drug is free of sedative effects, unless propranolol ultimately proves to be the exception. The converse is not true; stimulation is not equivalent to antidepressant effect. The most stimulant antidepressant, dextroamphetamine, is the one least well regarded clinically; the most sedative antidepressant, amitriptyline, is also the most highly regarded. The confusion between stimulation and antidepressant effect has even led some clinicians to deny the evidence of their senses and refer to tricyclic antidepressants as "energizers." The fact that drugs of this type may be both antidepressant and sedative has recently been exploited. One new tricyclic, doxepin, is widely promoted as effective both for anxiety and depression; the same assertion could be made for its close chemical relative, amitriptyline, which is equally sedative but more potent as an antidepressant.

In view of these considerations, it is hardly surprising that attempts to combine drugs such as amitriptyline and chlordiazepoxide have generally failed to advance the therapeutic efficacy, as compared with amitriptyline alone (74). Increasing evidence suggests that with the exception of those specific types of depressions mentioned above which are responsive to amitriptyline, the combination would rank no better than chlordiazepoxide alone. Drugs of the latter type are effective for many depressions with attendant symptoms of anxiety.

Antipsychotics and Antidepressants

The initial goal in combining these two classes of drugs was to "activate" withdrawn, retarded and possibly depressed schizophrenic patients who had not responded adequately to antipsychotics alone. Isocarboxazide, imipramine and the dextroamphetamine-amobarbital combinations were added to an established maintenance dose of chlorpromazine in carefully selected patients of this type (32). Not only did they not show any improvement, but those treated with dextroamphetamine-amobarbital combination became somewhat worse mentally and failed to show the weight gain of others. The combination of tranylcypromine and trifluoperazine was extensively studied and was marketed in several countries other than the United States for treating schizophrenic patients. For the most part, results indicated that the combination offered no more than the single drug, although the combination did not seem to be especially hazardous (203). Later, the hazards of tranylcypromine became more widely appreciated. With its decline as an antidepressant, use of this combination in treating schizophrenics also fell off.

The combination of perphenazine and amitriptyline was of considerable interest in that, while the effects of the component drugs were not enhanced, neither were they attenuated. Thus, schizophrenics treated with the combination did precisely as well as a previous group treated with perphenazine alone (99). A concurrent comparison subsequently confirmed this observation. Later on, when the combination was studied in a ratio more suitable for depressed patients, the same phenomenon prevailed. The combination was generally as good as the amitriptyline alone. With the further recognition that some depressions respond better to a phenothiazine and others to a tricyclic, the combination was found to be a useful all-around antidepressant, being equally effective at both sides of the spectrum, but no better than the properly chosen single drug (103). Thus, it appeared that this combination might be suitable for treating patients whose diagnosis might be in doubt, as between withdrawn schizophrenia or psychotic depression, or in whom the diagnostic subtype of depression might not be clinically apparent. It had the further advantage that the anticholinergic effects of amitriptyline afforded excellent protection against the extrapyramidal effects induced by perphenazine.

Other Combinations

Another possible way in which the effects of tricyclics might be enhanced would be to increase the sensitivity of receptors to the action of norepinephrine. This line of reasoning has been applied to the combined use of triiodothyronine and imipramine in treating depressions (234). Thyroid hormones, through mechanisms still not clear, are believed to sensitize the receptor sites for endogenous catecholamines. Thus, many of the symptoms of thyrotoxicosis resemble those from an infusion of epinephrine.

The presumption made for the combined treatment program is that central noradrenergic synapses are sensitized in a fashion similar to peripheral adrenergic receptor sites. Thus far, the evidence from the single group which has done the most work with this combination indicates increasing limitations on its value. Work from two independent sources has reached contradictory conclusions, one supporting the efficacy of the combination, the other failing to find it of value (62). As yet, it must be considered to be an experimental maneuver not to be widely adopted clinically.

We have already mentioned the use of combinations of an antipsychotic, such as perphenazine, with a tricyclic antidepressant, such as amitriptyline. The recent discovery that some antipsychotics may impair the metabolism of the tricyclics could enhance the value of the latter drug (but no more than might additional doses). On the other hand, one might assume that the antipsychotic, by blocking access of amines to their postsynaptic receptors, would attenuate the action of the tricyclics. The fact that in the clinic neither potentiation or attenuation ensues suggests that both mechanisms cancel each other out.

The use of methylphenidate to block the metabolism of tricyclic antidepressants again scarcely accomplishes more than simply giving larger doses of the latter drugs. Only if a pharmacological interaction between the drugs occurred as well would this combination provide a better treatment.

EXPERIMENTAL DRUG THERAPY OF DEPRESSION

Prior to the advent of effective antidepressant drugs, attempts had already begun to treat depressions with hallucinogens. LSD, initially administered to 25 ug doses with weekly or biweekly increments to 100 to 150 ug was given to twenty-nine patients with depressive states or borderline schizophrenic reactions. The number of treatments averaged five, ranging from one to sixteen. Improvement was noted in sixteen of twenty-two patients who could be followed for from six to seventeen months. Daily doses of 20 to 100 ug orally for one month were given to fifteen patients with psychotic depressions. Three recovered, four improved, four were unchanged, and four did not complete treatment. It was concluded that LSD offered no advantage over usual methods for treating depression (202).

Single doses of Ditran produced recovery of sixteen of twenty-five depressed patients given single doses of 10 to 20 mg, usually 15 mg, orally. Five relapsed during a follow-up period of three months, but the remainder maintained their remissions (15). Such reports as these indicate that a further look at this drug for treating depression is in order. It is of some interest that marihuana-like preparations were used in the past to treat depressions and one might anticipate that renewed attempts will be made with the newer preparations now available.

Another old idea which has been revived for use in treating depressions exploits the euphoriant effects of opiates or opioids. A combination of dextroamphetamine and meperidine in doses of 10 mg and 50 mg respectively was given intramuscularly three times during the first week, twice in the second week, to a maximum of six doses. Some beneficial effects were said to occur (139). Another old drug which has a reputation as an antidepressant is cocaine. According to present knowledge, it would be expected to work in a more potent but similar manner to amphetamines.

Levodopa, as a precursor both to dopamine and norepinephrine, might be expected to be an effective antidepressant, especially for those patients whose type of depression might fit the catecholamine hypothesis. Early results with this treatment were reported to be encouraging, especially in the retarded, endogenous type of depressed patient for whom it might be presumed to be most likely to be effective (25). My own experience at the same time, while treating five patients with levodopa, led me to consider it a completely ineffective treatment, which actually tended to elicit psychotic symptoms in patients who had not previously shown these. At present, there is little remaining enthusiasm for levodopa as an antidepressant and with increasing use of the drug in Parkinson's disease, it seems quite as likely to elicit a depression as to ameliorate it. Of course, we now know that large doses of levodopa, while raising brain concentrations of dopamine, have little effect on levels of norepinephrine and deplete concentrations of serotonin. The latter action might be related to its aggravation of depression in some patients.

Phobic anxiety associated with depression has been reported to be helped by the MAO inhibitor, phenelzine, either with or without a concomitant antianxiety drug. On the other hand, some cases of apparent anxiety reactions which are relieved by MAO inhibitors have been proposed as instances of "masked depression" (180).

SIDE EFFECTS AND COMPLICATIONS

Therapeutic Doses

Many of the side effects of antidepressants are extensions of their pharmacological actions. The dry mouth or blurred vision produced by the peripheral anticholinergic actions of tricyclics may be managed by such simple expedients as hard candy or magnifying lenses. More serious side effects, such as urinary retention or paralytic ileus, require immediate medical attention. One may often think that a formerly depressed patient is really psychotic when he merely suffers a toxic delirium due to the treatment. Just as with the phenothiazines, tricyclic antidepressants have been reported to cause cholestatic jaundice and agranulocytosis. Both of these complications are rare, and were never as frequent with these drugs as with the high-dose phenothiazines, quite possibly because tricyclics are seldom used for as long or in as high a dose.

The cardiac abnormalities produced by tricyclics are becoming matters of increasing concern. These drugs deplete the myocardium of catecholamines by preventing their uptake. Nonspecific T-wave changes somewhat similar to those from some phenothiazines are seen in many patients. Disturbances of cardiac rhythm and conduction are frequent complications of overdoses. Recently, cardiac standstill was found in a patient who had previously pretreated with guanethidine (232). The lowering of blood pressure produced by these drugs could be due to a combination of peripheral adrenergic blocking action as well as a decreased inotropic action on the heart.

The unexpected interactions of the MAOI and a number of

other drugs and foods have been extensively reviewed elsewhere (19). The clinical picture is one of an acute adrenergic crisis, similar to attacks associated with pheochromocytomas and for the same reason: increased amount of circulating norepinephrine. Nervous system signs include headache, stiff neck, nausea and vomiting and sometimes, subarachnoid hemorrhage. Cardiovascular signs include tachycardia, marked hypertension, and possibly acute pulmonary edema. The treatment of these reactions is like that of attacks of pheochromocytomas; phentolamine, 5 mg intravenously would be the preferred drug. Chlorpromazine would be a reasonable alternative for intramuscular injection.

As MAOI are also used for treating hypertension, they, too, may produce orthostatic hypotension in patients who are being treated for depression. One might expect these drugs would aggravate hypertension, but it is presumed that the hypotensive effect is due to formation of a false adrenergic transmitter, octopamine, which is considerably less active than norepinephrine. The latter is still the pressor agent of choice for any severe hypotensive reaction to these drugs.

Toxic Doses

It would be quite fitting if drugs used for treating depressed patients, where suicide is an ever-present danger, should be as safe as the antipsychotics. Unfortunately, this is not the case. As the problems from overdoses of tricyclics are different from those of MAO inhibitors, they will be discussed separately (106).

Doses of imipramine or amitriptyline in excess of 1.2 gm are seriously toxic with fatalities in adults fairly common after ingestion of 2.5 gm or more. Amitriptyline may be somewhat more toxic than imipramine and their demethylated metabolites somewhat less so. Whether these differences represent differences in the degree of central nervous system depression is still not certain. A decreasing level of consciousness leading to coma is regularly observed; early this may be preceeded by agitation or delirium. Cardiorespiratory depression with hypotension is frequent. Pupils are dilated and sluggish. Hyperthermia tends to occur. Myoclonic seizures, twitches, increased deep tendon reflexes and even plantar extensor responses are frequent concomitants of overdosage. The major distinguishing feature is a number of disturbances of cardiac rhythm and conduction. These include ventricular flutter or runs of tachcardia, atrial fibrillation or tachycardia, and varying degrees of atrioventricular or intraventricular block. These arrhythmias may be due to combined vagal block and a negative chronotropic effect.

The cardiac problems are uniquely difficult to manage. One is faced with controlling arrhythmias in the face of impaired cardiac conduction; as most commonly used drugs for control of arrhythmias would aggravate the conduction disturbances, it is probably better to avoid their use. The anticholinesterases, especially pyridostigmine or physostigmine, have been effective in diminishing toxicity in animals treated with toxic doses of amitriptyline. It is possible that these drugs might ameliorate some of the arrhythmias, as well as mental symptoms; doses of 0.5–1.0 mg intramuscularly have been recommended, with a repetition in 10 minutes if the pulse rate is not slowed. Electric cardioversion is a technique to be considered in the face of persistent arrhythmias. Because of the possibility of rapid changes in cardiac rhythm or cardiac arrest, continual EKG monitoring is desirable, with provisions at hand for defibrillation and resuscitation.

Treatment is in most respects similar to that outlined for the phenothiazines. In the most severely intoxicated patient to recover, mannitol was used as an osmotic diuretic to hasten excretion of drug, and dialysis was used to manage hyperpyrexia. More than with the phenothiazines, the tricyclic antidepressants tend to induce bladder and bowel paralysis due to their strong anticholinergic effects. Just as with phenothiazines, the potentiation of sedative effects of barbiturates makes these drugs less preferable than others for managing seizures. It should be remembered that one of the pharmacological tests for compounds of this type is the potentiation of pressor responses to norepinephrine; use of pressor amines should be considered only if plasma expanders and fluid replacement fail to alleviate shock.

Just as with phenothiazines, removal of these drugs prior to absorption is easy but extremely difficult after they have been bound to protein. There is little evidence that these drugs are dialyzable, so the excretory route of choice is by forced diuresis.

A 500 mg dose (fifty 10 mg tablets) of tranylcypromine proved fatal for a 17-year-old girl who exhibited agitation, delirium, tremors, sweating, coma, shock, heart block, and profound hyperthermia (110°) for eight hours before she died. Barbiturates were used, but were ineffective; a slight fall in body temperature was achieved by tubbing. A 15-year-old girl who ingested 350 mg of tranycypromine was subjected to hemodialysis and made a rapid recovery; presumably the drug can be dialyzed readily. Ingestion of a dose of 750 (fifty 15 mg tablets) of phenelzine was not fatal in a patient weighing 54 kg, but ataxia, weakness, drowsiness, delirium, seizures, muscle fasciculations, and hyperthermia were encountered. Administration of CPZ appeared to be an effective antagonist. That the latter drug was effective seems reasonable, for most of the toxic effects of the MAO inhibitors are attributable to excessive adrenergic stimulation. In this regard, toxicity of these drugs resembles that from amphetamines. Reports of overdoses of these drugs are still infrequent; one would hope that this is due to their declining use. Many of us believe that the lack of convincing evidence for efficacy of these drugs in controlled trials in depressed patients, as well as their hazards, contraindicate their use.

SUMMARY

Depression may be the most common disorder which psychiatrists must treat. It is one of the few that may be lethal. Anxiety is almost always a concomitant symptom. The clinical manifestations of depression may take the form of several syndromes, possibly differing in their etiology. Endogenous depressions are the most severe and probably have a genetic-biochemical basis. These depressions fortunately respond best to tricyclic antidepressant drugs. Other types of depressions may either require no specific drug treatment, or may be better managed with other drugs, including antianxiety drugs, small doses of phenothiazines, or stimulants. Concurrent treatment with psychotherapy, or in severe cases, with electroconvulsive therapy, is required for optimum outcome. Doses of antidepressants should be carefully monitored to meet each patient's needs. Duration of treatment depends on the natural history of depression in each patient. Despite the controversy which surrounds antidepressant drugs, they are useful when given for the proper indications.

CHAPTER 5

ANTIANXIETY DRUGS

 $\rm A$ NTIANXIETY drugs are widely used, some might say over-used, in the clinical practice of medicine. In the United States the use of such drugs continues to increase with each passing year, the total use having doubled in the last several years. Whether the increase is the result of the generally turbulent times which have prevailed in the past decade, or the introduction of new drugs and their widespread promotion, or of sloppy prescribing practices of physicians is uncertain.

Despite their wide popularity, antianxiety drugs continue to be controversial (194). Many assert that such great dependence on drug therapy for symptoms that seem to be rooted in life experience may deny patients the benefits of other treatments. Although the efficacy of these drugs for relieving symptoms of anxiety is generally accepted, the difficulties in showing differences between active drugs and placebos make many doubt that the benefits of drug therapy are very great. Finally, the rapid increase of nonmedical use of mind-altering drugs has led to concerns that overenthusiastic prescribing of these drugs may contribute to this problem.

ANXIETY – UBIQUITOUS SYMPTOM

Most of us who work constantly against ever-pressing deadlines think we have some appreciation of anxiety. The frustration of running out of time or energy before all is accomplished, the uncertainty of many tasks started and still unfinished; and even the sense of failure imparted by the typical "examination" dream are fairly common experiences. Still, the effect of anxiety, which is so widely shared, may be integrated and handled within one's ordinary existence. Perhaps in mild forms anxiety may even be helpful; those who have "examination" dreams rarely fail.

Defining anxiety isn't easy, despite the fact that most of us will acknowledge a personal acquaintance with the symptoms of anxiety. Anxiety and fear can be readily distinguished: Fear is acute; the precipitating causes are real and recognized; the physiological responses are immediate and dramatic. In anxiety, the reaction is more chronic and attenuated, and usually the cause is not easily discernible. The predominant feeling is apprehension, often about some unspecified future threat. To varying degrees, such a feeling may be either so mildly unpleasant as to make us strive harder, or so unbearably painful as to hinder all productive effort. Anxious people often complain of feeling tense. The two words are not interchangeable: Anxiety is purely subjective, a symptom; tension is manifested objectively by a variety of signs.

ETIOLOGICAL CONSIDERATIONS

Anxiety is believed to be a reaction to a psychological stimulus, either from within or from outside. When external stimuli are clearly threatening, the subjective response is fear. The types of external stimuli that provoke anxiety are not overtly threatening but may symbolize stimuli associated from childhood with a threat.

If the stimuli come primarily from within and are triggered by external events, the response tends to be less intense than fear — and more chronic. Such anxiety is often called "free floating," and its causes may lie buried in the unconscious. In milder forms, such anxiety may produce the melange of symptoms with which patients frustrate physicians who seek some organic cause. In more severe forms, this type of anxiety can lead to the anguish with which the psychiatrist must deal.

The many symptoms of anxiety are attributable to the fact that, more than any other emotional stress, anxiety can induce widespread physiological changes. The Cannon hypothesis is still the explanation most widely held: Anxiety is perceived as a threat arising primarily from within, triggering somatic and visceral responses through the autonomic nervous system and the hypothalamic-pituitary-endocrine system. The James-Lange theory, that anxiety is perceived only after somatic or visceral responses have occurred, is less widely held but is enjoying a modest revival in this day of servomechanisms and feedback loops. The signal theory, proposed by Freud, is not too different: Some remembrance of a past threat, triggered by some unrecognized present situation, signals the feeling tone and somatic responses of the past fearful state. Nor is the theory of Hughlings Jackson much different; it postulates that the mental and somatic aspects coincide closely in time.

MANIFESTATIONS OF ANXIETY

Fatigue, dizziness, vague aches and pains, palpitations, headache, insomnia, irritability, indigestion — every bodily system can be affected, and the catalog of psychosomatic disorders, part of whose pathogenesis is believed to be anxiety, contains some of the most frequent ills that befall man: obesity, hypertension, asthma, irritable colon, peptic ulcer, eczema and other skin eruptions, cardiac neurosis, and hyperventilation syndrome. The etiologic role of anxiety in these conditions is still debatable, but there is little doubt that anxiety is prominent in them, as well as in a host of medical and surgical situations in which no etiologic role is claimed for anxiety.

Bodily symptoms may only be the more easily appreciated symptoms of anxiety. Behavioral changes are also pronounced, though more subtle. The patient whose frustration tolerance is low, who is irritable and easily upset, who is distractable and disinterested in his work, may be showing common manifestations of anxiety. Most cases of insomnia have anxiety or depression as their basis, more often than not, together. Anxiety may provoke excessive drinking, the sedative effects of alcohol being a kind of self-administered antianxiety drug. Schizophrenics are also commonly anxious, and many initially present for treatment with what appears to be an uncomplicated anxiety reaction. Thus, anxiety may be part of a great many abnormal emotional and behavioral disturbances. Such anxiety is what psychiatrists are commonly called upon to treat and it can be a severely disabling illness to the affected individual.

Thus, anxiety can be a symptom, a concomitant of other

physical illnesses, an illness in its own right, or associated with other more severe disturbances such as depression, alcoholism, and schizophrenia.

KINDS OF ANXIETY

The conceptualization of anxiety is rather complex, and is usually thought of in two major categories, anxiety which may vary as a personal characteristic and anxiety which may exist at a specific time dependent upon a number of variables. The former aspect of anxiety, often termed "characteristic," "trait" or "basic," includes both the "normal" level of anxiousness for a particular person as well as his susceptibility to anxiety under stressful provocations. Although this concept of anxiety has theoretical implications, it does not usually concern us in the clinic. We treat current anxiety.

It might very well be debated whether all current anxiety should be treated, but it seems clear that when anxiety is of a degree severe enough to cause dysfunction or discomfort, treatment is required. Few reasonable physicians would take the position that such anxiety should be treated solely by drugs or solely by psychotherapy. The case for non-drug treatment seems well established by abundant evidence that anxiety may result from unresolved intrapsychic conflicts or environmental stresses. To the extent that conflicts may be resolved or the environment improved, anxiety may be relieved. On the other hand, many clinical studies indicate that drug therapy may be effective in providing symptomatic relief, at least as compared with no drug therapy or with placebo. In fact, one of the best studies indicates that drugs may provide as much relief as psychotherapy (22). Obviously, the choice should not be "either/or" but "both."

PROBLEMS IN THE CLINICAL EVALUATION
OF ANTIANXIETY DRUGS

Measurement of Anxiety

Anxiety should be clearly distinguished from tension. Although the two symptoms may parallel each other, one is essentially subjective, the other objective. Thus, if we are to measure anxiety, we are pretty much at the mercy of what patients tell us, either by reporting on their symptoms and feelings without our intervention (self-reports) or with it (interviews). In the latter situation, it is not always possible, nor necessarily desirable, to separate anxiety from tension. The quavering voice, the wet armpits, the tremulous hands, the nervous tics of our patients should not escape our notice and are certainly relevant data. Most clinical scales, however, rely on subjective data (154).

One of the most widely used self-reporting anxiety scales is the IPAT (Institute for Personality and Ability Testing) or Scheier-Cattell scale (Schema II). This scale consists of 95 items, of which 30 correlate quite highly with anxiety levels. The patient indicates the degree of the individual item using a midpoint of zero and plus and minus to show positive or negative deviations from normal. Three points are given for a plus or minus response when appropriate, one point when these responses are inappropriate and two points for a zero response. The total score indicates the prevailing level of anxiety (33). A number of adjective checklists have been proposed, including the Mood Adjective Check List and the Multiple Affect Adjective Check List (241). In the latter, adjectives are positively or negatively related to anxiety; the positive items score one point if checked as present, the negative ones a point if checked as absent. Other scoring systems for such checklists use a three- or four-point scale.

The MMPI (Minnesota Multiphasic Personality Inventory) is a widely used self-report scale, from which has been derived a number of subscales especially suitable for rating anxiety. The Manifest Anxiety Scale is the most familiar of these, but others may be equally suitable (222). Ordinarily, self-report scales are quite suitable for patients with the predominant symptoms of anxiety (psychoneuroses, psychosomatic disorders, nervousness), but progressively less reliable in depression or psychoses.

Interview scales are equally suitable for measuring anxiety and can usually be accomplished within the context of a clinical interview, so that, unlike the self-report techniques, the patient may not even be aware that he is being rated. The Wittenborn

Psychiatric Rating Scale, which contains a number of anxiety-related items, can be used this way (235). The BPRS (Brief Psychiatric Rating Scale), while devised to cover a broad range of psychopathology, can also be used to codify global symptoms of anxiety, tension, somatic complaints and depression, each specifically relevant to the measurement of anxiety and its attendant phenomena (164). Finally, many improvised symptom-sign checklists have been devised which are usually quite suitable, although many of these ad hoc measurements have not been fully validated.

For purposes of a clinical study evaluating the efficacy of antianxiety drugs, other types of anxiety measurements are far less often used. While projective tests may be used to measure anxiety, their administration and interpretation is far more complex than the simpler clinical rating scales. Specialized techniques, such as verbal analysis, also have stringent clinical limitations. Physiological measurements of anxiety often leave much to be desired, in that they require special equipment and often elaborate procedures. One of the more impressive attempts combined clinical, psychological and physiological measurements of anxiety to compare chlordiazepoxide with placebo after a week of treatment (124). Chlordiazepoxide was significantly superior to placebo in observer and self-ratings of global improvement and depression and self-ratings of anxiety (clinical measurements), decreased dizzy factor score on the Clyde Mood Scale (psychological measurement), and decreased resting and basal forearm blood flow (physiological measurement). Comparing an active drug against placebo is much simpler than comparing two active drugs. Multiple measurements in the latter case frequently show differences in either direction.

Selection of Patients and Sample Size

One would think that anxious patients would be so abundant that there should be no problem in finding enough who were symptomatic so that adequate drug studies could be done. Just because patients are abundant, however, doesn't necessarily mean that they are most suitable. Many anxious patients seen in physicians' offices or clinics have chronic anxiety that has been reinforced by serious job, marital and alcohol problems, or concurrent medical illnesses. Most have already been exposed to a large variety of drugs, and the more well-to-do to some sort of psychotherapy. These patients are still the ones most often used for comparing antianxiety drugs, but when one delves closely into their social and medical problems, it seems almost unrealistic to expect them to show appreciable responses to drugs. Quite likely, many of the failures to distinguish antianxiety drugs from placebo stem from this source of negative bias.

Another reason for lack of sensitivity in distinguishing between drugs and placebo, or possibly between active drugs, is an insufficient sample size. As a general rule, the smaller the difference between treatments, the larger the sample size that is required for such differences to be statistically significant. Practical experience suggests that a sample size of at least 30 in each treatment group is reasonable, and that one should not miss differences of large degree given a reasonably homogeneous sample. If one has to treat 100 patients in each group to show a statistically significant difference, the actual difference involved may not be of clinical importance.

Experimental Designs

The great variations in the course of anxiety dictate the need for controlled studies wherever these are possible. Most studies of antianxiety drugs employ a chronic treatment regimen, which may vary from a few weeks to a few months, with fixed doses of drugs, the latter being randomly assigned. This type of experimental design may not be appropriate for antianxiety agents. An intriguing experimental design would be one in which drug treatments being tested would be employed for very limited periods on an ad hoc basis during separate episodes of anxiety. The assignment by episodes would be random, with an evaluation of relief being obtained for each episode. One might think in terms of treatment lasting no more than five to seven days and of dosage schedules which would emphasize using the major daily dose at bedtime and additional small doses during the day as needed. The treatment of successive episodes would have to be separated by no-treatment intervals of about equal length, but this procedure should not impose too great a hardship. Such a design might more closely reflect the use of these drugs in practice, and could conceivably lead to a clearer separation of efficacious drugs.

Other Methodological Approaches

Comparisons of antianxiety drugs in normal subjects are always open to the charge that the effect of major interest may be missed and that one only measures different degrees of impairment which are most likely artefacts of dose. This criticism seems valid in the light of two studies using film-provoked anxiety. College students given single doses of placebo, secobarbital, or chlordiazepoxide before viewing an anxiety-inducing film showed only sedative but not antianxiety effects from the drugs (172). A comparison of diazepam 20 mg daily with placebo in moderate to severe anxious patients indicated that the drug diminished several autonomic responses of anxiety induced by the film (35). Patients were more sensitive indicators of drug action than normal subjects, at least in this experimental situation.

In general, one might say that present clinical techniques for evaluating antianxiety drugs leave much to be desired, just as do the techniques of animal pharmacological screening.

CHEMICAL CLASSES AND PHARMACOLOGICAL PROPERTIES

A wide array of drugs claim efficacy for treating anxiety (135). On the one hand are those drugs which possess varying degrees of the pharmacological actions of sedative-hypnotics. They depress the central nervous system to various degrees dependent upon dosage, milder depression often resulting in the desired therapeutic effect, relief of anxiety, along with some degree of impairment of various psychological functions, while larger doses may enforce sleep, and toxic doses produce deep coma. Many of these drugs are anticonvulsant by virtue of depression of the motor cortex. Block of spinal cord internuncial neurones, as well as the sedative effects, contributes to a muscle relaxant action; overdoses of most are manifested by weakness, incoordination, and flaccidity. The development of tolerance on repeated use, as well as the tendency of some persons to abuse these drugs, may lead to physical dependence manifested by withdrawal reactions on abrupt discontinuation. In these respects, most of the newer antianxiety agents share pharmacological properties of the barbiturates, although in varying degrees.

On the other hand are drugs which might be termed "sedative-autonomic," which unlike the others, affect the peripheral autonomic nervous system. They also differ in increasing muscle tone, lowering convulsive thresholds and lacking the potential for habituation and physical dependence. Drugs in this class include sedative antihistaminics, such as hydroxyzine or diphenhydramine, phenothiazine antipsychotics, and the more sedative tricyclic antidepressants, such as doxepin or amitriptyline (See Fig. 5-1).

Most clinicians, as well as patients, prefer drugs of the sedative-hypnotic type. Their sedation is more familiar to us, resembling that of alcohol. The sedative-autonomic drugs often create feelings of inner restlessness and mental fuzziness, as well as having bothersome side effects, such as dry mouth or blurred vision. These same effects make such drugs unlikely choices for drugs of abuse, but less acceptable therapeutic agents. Still, some patients tolerate the side effects and gain more therapeutic benefit from these drugs than the other group (80).

Animal pharmacologists may complain, not without reason, about such a simple classification of these drugs. Special exception may be taken to grouping together such drugs as phenobarbital, meprobamate and the benzodiazepines, without taking into account the many differences that have been found in various pharmacological tests (16, 113, 189). The key phrase "varying degrees" is an adequate qualifier, at least in describing those pharmacological differences of clinical importance. One can get into many arguments about the various similarities and differences among the pharmacological properties of sedative-hypnotic anti-anxiety drugs, but to the clinician the similarities outweigh the differences, with exceptions to be noted below.

To a considerable extent, these resemblances may be an artefact

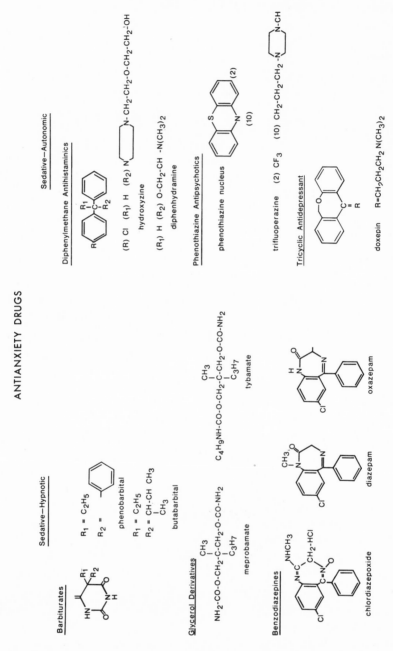

Figure 5-1. Structural relationship between various antianxiety drugs.

of the animal pharmacological screening tests used for detecting potential antianxiety drugs. Diminution of spontaneous activity, prolongation of hexobarbital sleeping time, increased seizure threshold, hind-limb ataxia and many other animal tests clearly employ the barbiturate model. Little wonder that most other drugs resemble them. In fact, it seems doubtful that a truly differenty type of antianxiety drug would have passed the usual pre-clinical screening tests. If propranolol proves to be an effective antianxiety agent, as preliminary evidence suggests, it will be necessary to take a searching look at many of the traditional screening tests for antianxiety drugs (84). So far as we can tell at the moment, all drugs effective against anxiety are central nervous system depressants, with the possible exception just mentioned.

METABOLISM AND PHARMACOKINETICS

Phenobarbital, being a free acid, is absorbed somewhat slowly. Its binding to plasma and brain proteins is comparatively low, so its onset of action is further slowed (208). The drug has a long persistence in plasma once a steady-state condition is attained. Hydroxylation is the major route for metabolism of phenobarbital. About 30 percent of the drug is excreted unchanged in the urine, which is the greatest renal excretion of unmetabolized drug of any barbiturate. Thus, phenobarbital might be a preferred drug in cases of hepatic impairment but should best be avoided in cases of renal impairment. Although phenobarbital is established as an extremely potent inducer of drug-metabolizing enzymes, including those for its own metabolism, metabolic tolerance to the effects of the drug in man seem to be far less important than pharmaco-dynamic tolerance. The slow rate of absorption and disappearance time of the drug make it an unlikely candidate for abuse or for the production of severe withdrawal reactions.

Meprobamate is rapidly absorbed when given orally, with peak levels probably being attained in 3 to 4 hours after a single dose. The disappearance rate from plasma is fairly rapid with a T½ ranging from six to sixteen hours with a mean of about eleven hours following single doses (102). Meprobamate is hydroxylated in the liver. The ratio of hydroxylated drug to free drug in urine is low after a single dose, but increases rapidly with chronic administration, doubling within a week. Thus, like phenobarbital, meprobamate stimulates its own metabolism. In the latter case, metabolic tolerance is more appreciable clinically, possibly because of the much shorter persistence of meprobamate in plasma. The meprobamate homolog, tybamate, shows both erratic absorption and an extremely rapid plasma disappearance rate. The calculated T½ of this drug is about six hours. These two attributes are somewhat disadvantageous clinically. On the other hand, it is virtually impossible to sustain a high enough concentration in plasma to produce a withdrawal reaction (209).

Chlordiazepoxide is readily but not rapidly absorbed. Therapeutic doses produce steady-state concentrations in a few days, usually with plasma levels in the range of 3 to 8 ug/ml. The plasma T½ is rather long, being estimated at 24 to 36 hours following single doses and 48 hours following chronic doses (97). Very little chlordiazepoxide is excreted in the urine, about 1 to 2 percent as unchanged drug and about 3 to 6 percent as conjugated drug. Two pharmacologically active metabolites are formed, a lactam form and a free amine form (See Fig. 5-2). Following therapeutic doses of 40 mg daily for 14 days, plasma concentrations of chlordiazepoxide were 2 ug/ml; of the lactam, 1 ug/ml; and of the amine, 1 ug/ml. The long persistence of active drug and metabolites makes chlordiazepoxide an unlikely drug for abuse (189).

Diazepam is absorbed more rapidly than chlordiazepoxide. The initial decline in plasma concentrations is rapid, followed by a much longer slow phase, which results in accumulation of drug with repeated doses. Diazepam forms several metabolites, oxydesmethyldiazepam being active enough to be used as a drug in its own right. With chronic doses, both diazepam and desmethyldiazepam accumulate, reaching a steady state in four and five days, respectively. The estimated plasma T½ following subchronic doses is 20 to 42 hours for diazepam and 42 to 96 hours for desmethyldiazepam (225). Diazepam is about 96 percent protein-bound in plasma. It distributes rapidly to brain and body fat in animals, being slowly released from the latter depot. Evidence of gastric secretion or enterohepatic cycling of the drug may provide even more basis for its prolonged clinical action. The

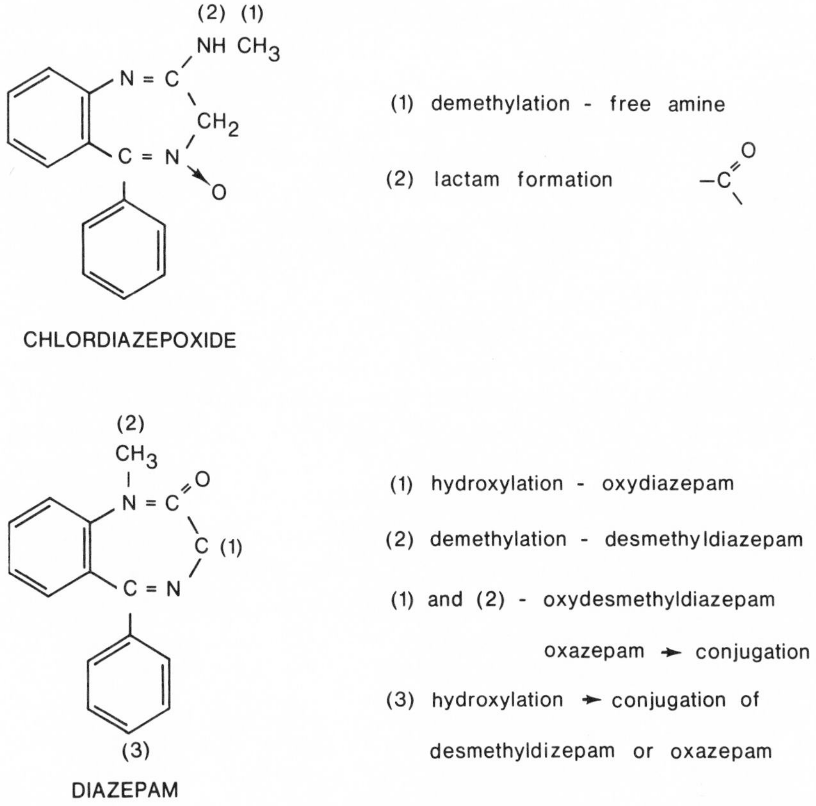
(2) (1)
NH CH3
N = C
CH2
C = N
O
CHLORDIAZEPOXIDE
(1) demethylation - free amine
(2) lactam formation
(2)
CH3
N = C
O
C (1)
C = N
(3)
DIAZEPAM
(1) hydroxylation - oxydiazepam
(2) demethylation - desmethyldiazepam
(1) and (2) - oxydesmethyldiazepam
oxazepam → conjugation
(3) hydroxylation → conjugation of
desmethyldizepam or oxazepam

Figure 5-2. Metabolism of chlordiazepoxide and diazepam. Formation ot active metabolites may account for long clinical duration of effects.

drug passes readily through the placenta, as measured by autoradiographic techniques (112). Although both chlordiazepoxide and diazepam can induce drug-metabolizing enzymes, they do not appear to be as potent in this regard as the drugs mentioned above (119). They do not tend to appreciably increase their own metabolism, or if they do, the production of active metabolites seems to eliminate the possibility of a clinically meaningful degree of metabolic tolerance.

EFFICACY IN ANXIETY

Considering the widespread and continuing use of these drugs, it may seem impertinent to question their efficacy. Yet a number of well-designed controlled studies have failed to show consistent differences between drug and placebo therapy of anxiety. The negative biases provided by a poor sample or an insufficient sample size have already been mentioned. Fixed doses of drugs and fixed durations of treatment may also contribute negative bias. One of the better studies of doxepin as an antianxiety drug compared it with diazepam and placebo in a large group of anxious post-alcoholic patients (72). At the end of four weeks of treatment, no significant differences were found between the treatments. One would expect that anxiety would be even more transitory in this group of patients than in most, so that a briefer course of treatment might have been more sensitive to specific effects of drug as contrasted with the natural course of the symptom. Such was the case, for the comparisons made at one week showed both drugs to be better than placebo, a finding given no emphasis by the investigators. Probably most important in making it difficult to distinguish drug effects in anxious patients are the large number of metapharmacological factors, involving the patient, the physician and the setting of treatment which may interact with the pharmacological effects of drugs and placebo.

Difficulties in showing differences between drugs and placebos in treating anxiety are recurrent. A large-scale study of chronically anxious male veterans revealed no differences in responses to meprobamate, chlorpromazine, phenobarbital, or placebo when added to a program of psychotherapy. Phenobarbital tended to make the patients somewhat worse (141). Subsequent studies of the same group indicated that chlordiazepoxide and placebo both produced more improvement than was found in a no-drug group regardless of whether or not concurrent psychotherapy was given. After the first week, patients receiving the drug were somewhat better than the placebo-treated patients, but no differences were noted at the end of four weeks (142). A later study indicated that chlordiazepoxide was somewhat better than meprobamate and placebo in similar patients, although the differences were more apparent in this case after four to six weeks of treatment (153). Anxious patients treated with meprobamate, prochlorperazine, and phenobarbital, along with brief clinic visits, did no better (or

any worse) than those treated with placebo or weekly psychotherapy of one hour's duration. All treatment groups improved
more than a no-treatment group. The meprobamate and psychotherapy groups were slightly more improved than the others; least
improvement was noted in those treated with phenobarbital or
prochlorperazine (22). Thus several problems soon became
evident: anxious patients tend to respond favorably to any
attention, including placebo; differences between drugs and
placebos are often subtle and transient; drugs, but not placebos,
may interact with nonsepcific factors in the treatment situation
such as the personality of the physician.

These difficulties have continued to plague investigators.
Diazepam, even in doses up to 40 mg daily, was no more effective
than placebo in treating anxious outpatients (88). The major
problem in this study was the rather high (55%) improvement rate
among the placebo-treated patients. Even when treatment periods
were limited to one to two weeks, it was difficult to show the
superiority of oxazepam over placebo in psychiatric outpatients,
although a number of indicators favored the latter drug (115). In
this study, the sample size was probably too small to show any but
a major difference, something not too likely to occur in this area
of treatment. The authors questioned whether rating devices for
measuring change in neurotic patients were as sensitive as those
used in rating psychotic patients. An alternative explanation might
be that the changes produced by antipsychotic drugs are much
larger in a disorder not so prone to rapid spontaneous remission.

Considering these difficulties, more weight must be given to
studies which have demonstrated differences between treatments.
Meprobamate (1,600 mg per day), prochlorperazine (20 mg per
day), amobarbital sodium (120 mg per day) and placebo were
compared in psychoneurotic outpatients. During the first two
weeks of treatment, all were equally effective, but the three drugs
surpassed placebo on the subsequent two-week trials in a crossover
design (191). This finding − that the initial treatment used is often
efficacious, regardless of what it is − has been a recurring theme in
antianxiety drug studies. Another study by the same group
compared meprobamate (1,600 mg per day) with phenobarbital
sodium (60 mg per day) and placebo, in both medical and

psychiatric clinic patients. Interestingly, the degree of anxiety present in patients influenced the results. Meprobamate was better than the other two treatments in the mildly to moderately anxious patients; phenobarbital appeared to be superior in the highly anxious patients. Over a series of studies involving neurotic outpatients, it was found that diazepam (15 mg per day) was preferred over chlordiazepoxide (30 mg per day) which in turn was preferred to amobarbital sodium (150 mg per day) (117). That it should be possible to distinguish between diazepam and chlordiazepoxide seems strange, for they are virtually identical in their spectrum of pharmacological actions except for potency. Another group also found diazepam (15 mg per day) superior to amobarbital sodium (180 mg per day) in alleviating symptoms of anxiety. A comparison of oxazepam and chlordiazepoxide in various types of anxious outpatients did not demonstrate any special advantage of oxazepam in terms of rapidity of action or overall effectiveness (73). Difficulties in detecting differences between similar types of psychotherapeutic drugs are not limited to antianxiety drugs by any means, but the difficulties are somewhat greater.

Frequently tabulations summarize the results of blind, controlled comparisons between various antianxiety drugs: In so many studies, drug A was better than placebo; and in so many it was not; in so many studies, drug A was better than drug B; and in so many studies it was equal to drug B; and in so many it was inferior to drug B. Such tabulations make the assumption that all blind controlled trials are equally valid, which is often clearly not the case. When one considers the clinical evidence to date, one is inclined to rank the benzodiazepines ahead of meprobamate and phenobarbital, and them in turn, ahead of placebo. Nonetheless, some might question whether or not the rank order can be that clearly defined; one review of the comparative studies of chlordiazepoxide and amobarbital sodium concluded that except for differences in potency, the drugs were approximately equally efficacious (133). On the other hand, another group found diazepam (15 mg per day) superior to amobarbital sodium (180 mg per day) in alleviating anxiety (152).

Under such conditions, it is always hazardous to make the

assumption that because no significant difference was found between two drugs, they must necessarily be equally effective. A provocative comparison of chlordiazepoxide (30 mg per day) and propranolol (90 mg per day) concluded that they were equally effective in treating anxiety, but that chlordiazepoxide was better for treating symptoms of depression and sleep disturbance. Sedative side effects were greater with chlordiazepoxide (231). Although some evidence is accumulating that propranolol has antianxiety actions, it may be premature to conclude that it is the equal of all the current drugs. Given all the confounding variables implicit in distinguishing drugs of this class, it is most unlikely that differences between two active agents will be found unless a very large sample size is employed. One will have failed to reject the null hypothesis when one should have. Such a danger exists in regard to evaluations of other types of psychotherapeutic drugs as well. Thus, one must guard against committing the "not significantly different from, therefore equal to" fallacy.

EFFICACY IN DEPRESSION

Quite early, meprobamate was reported to be helpful in some depressed patients. A controlled comparison of meprobamate, protriptyline, a combination of the two drugs, and placebo indicated that patients improved significantly more after receiving the three drug treatments than after the placebo (192). More recent use of benzodiazepines, such as diazepam in depressions, also suggested therapeutic benefits. The most recent study of consequence compared acetophenazine with diazepam in patients diagnosed as "anxious depressions" (109). Previous studies by this group had established that phenothiazines were preferable to tricyclics in this most frequent type of depressive reaction. As both groups were equally improved in the latest study, it was concluded that benzodiazepines were also effective and were probably preferred over the more hazardous phenothiazines.

METAPHARMACOLOGICAL CONSIDERATIONS

Some of the difficulty in making an accurate appraisal of

antianxiety drugs is due to placebo effects. Anxious patients tend to respond favorably to any attention, including placebo; differences between drugs and placebos are often subtle and transient; drugs, but not placebos, may interact with nonspecific factors in the treatment situation, such as the personality of the physician. In a study that has become something of a classic, meprobamate was compared with placebo in anxious patients, using all the customary criteria of a double blind controlled study, but adding the variable of having two different physicians doing the prescribing. One physician was trained to take a "therapeutic ʼstance; he was generally supportive and sympathetic and had great confidence in the treatment. The other took an "experimental" stance, with somewhat opposite attitudes. The difference between drug and placebo was significant in the group of patients treated by the first physician, but not in those patients treated by the second (223). The moral is clear: If you are going to prescribe these drugs, at least try to work up some enthusiasm for them and try to communicate it to your patients.

The patient's personality may also contribute to his response to drugs. Patients with personality characteristics of extroversion and being physically active ("doers") tend to respond to antianxiety drugs with an increase in anxiety. Presumably, any drug that interfered in any way with their will to achieve, or their ability to handle anxiety by physical movement, actually made things worse. On the other hand, such drugs seemed to be well tolerated and beneficial for patients who were intellectual, passive, and esthetically inclined ("thinkers"). Thus, it seems possible that some failures in the use of antianxiety drugs may be attributed to their immobilizing one of the defenses against anxiety used by a particular type of personality. Such patients might be better treated with much smaller doses of drug than are customarily used, or possibly without such drugs at all.

In addition to these two readily identifiable factors that influence responses to antianxiety drugs, many others have also been detected in the prescribing physician (his general belief in the efficacy of drugs as compared with other treatments), the patient (his initial level of anxiety, his degree of "squareness," his expectations from psychiatric treatment, and his past personal experience with drugs), and the treatment setting (results are better in charity clinics than in private psychiatric practice, with general practitioners getting results in the middle). Not all these considerations can be exploited to increase the efficacy of treatment, but some can be good indicators of what one might expect from drug therapy in a given patient treated by a given physician in a given setting of treatment (193).

Nonspecific factors which may influence the action of the drug constantly nag the clinical psychopharmacologist. When one deals with drugs which alter awareness, consciousness and subjective feelings, such influences as the expectation of the patient (or his physician), the setting in which the drug is given, and the subsequent reinforcements of the results of drug therapy influence the outcome. On the other hand, the more effective a drug is or the more serious the disorder being treated, the less likely these effects will be confounding. As Max Hamilton put it: "Nonspecific factors are important for small treatments and small illnesses." Consequently, we are more plagued by these variables in the case of evaluating antianxiety drugs than we are in evaluating antipsychotics. But psychopharmacologists are not alone: Cardiologists might have far less difficulty identifying a truly effective treatment for cardiogenic shock than they have in trying to determine the efficacy of antianginal drugs.

CHOICE OF ANTIANXIETY DRUG

The extensive popularity of the benzodiazepines may stem from a few important pharmacological differences (See Table 5-I).

First, and most important, the benzodiazepines are virtually suicide-proof. Massive overdoses have been taken with very little difficulty in managing patients and no fatalities in the absence of other drugs (51). The safety of benzodiazepines is probably related to less depression of the neurogenic respiratory drive than with conventional sedative-hypnotic drugs. This same advantage is also found with the phenothiazines.

Second, metabolic tolerance to the benzodiazepines is a lesser problem than it is with meprobamate, or with phenobarbital, both of which rapidly induce their own drug-metabolizing enzymes

Clinical Use of Psychotherapeutic Drugs

Table 5-I

Differential Pharmacological Properties of Antianxiety Drugs

	Pb	*Mep*	*Benz*	*Diph*	*Pheno*	*Tri*
Antianxiety/sedative ratio	+	++	++	$\underline{+}$	$\underline{+}$	$\underline{+}$
Muscle relaxation	$\underline{+}$	++	+++	0	$\underline{-}$	0
Anticonvulsant action	+++	++	+++	$\underline{-}$	$\underline{-}$	$\underline{-}$
Duration of action	+++	+	+++	+	++	++
Tolerance	++	+++	+	0	0	0
Habituation	$\underline{+}$	+++	$\underline{+}$	0	0	0
Physical dependence	+	+++	+	0	0	0
Disturbed sleep pattern	++	++	$\underline{+}$	++	++	++
Potential suicidal use	++	+++	0	++	0	+++

Signs indicate degree or probability, ranging from (−) opposite effect, (0) none, ($\underline{+}$) minimal, (+) slight, (++) moderate, (+++) great
Pb − phenobarbital; Mep − glycerol derivatives; Benz − denzodiazepines; Diph − diphenylmethane antihistaminics; Pheno − phenothiazines; Tri − tricyclics

(40). Although pharmacodynamic, or behavioral tolerance, does not appear to be a great clinical problem with the other two drugs (consider the sustained anticonvulsant effects of phenobarbital taken chronically), it is probably minimal with the benzodiazepines. Thus, the latter drugs are less likely to lose their clinical effects on chronic dosage, requiring greater amounts to sustain remission.

Third, the duration of action of the benzodiazepines is somewhat longer than that of meprobamate. Most benzodiazepines have plasma half-lives in man of 24 to 48 hours, while that of meprobamate is around 12 hours (102, 189). A prolonged duration of action is desirable in that doses need be less frequent, and that clinical benefits are more sustained. In this regard, the benzodiazepines resemble phenobarbital, which also persists for a long while.

Fourth, the relative lack of tolerance to the drug and long duration of action makes it a poor candidate for production of physical dependence. Physical dependence to chlordiazepoxide occurs, but only with extremes of dose and duration of treatment

(98). Because of its prolonged sojourn in the body, chlordiazepoxide does not produce the immediate, severe type of withdrawal reaction which follows abrupt discontinuation of meprobamate. Presumably, this reaction is related in part to the rapidity of declines of plasma and tissue concentrations of drug. Over the years, it has been difficult to find well-documented cases of withdrawal reaction associated with clinical use of benzodiazepines. To some extent, the same is true for phenobarbital which, while as available in the black market as secobarbital sodium, is far less favored as a drug of abuse.

Finally, a number of studies from various sleep laboratories indicate that benzodiazepines produce remarkably little change in normal sleep patterns as compared with most other sedative-hypnotic drugs. As it may be highly desirable to exploit the hypnotic effects of antianxiety drugs. one would like to minimize alterations in normal sleep patterns. Nonetheless, benzodiazepines consistently decrease the amount of time spent in slow-wave sleep, so that until the consequences of this change in sleep pattern is elucidated, their chronic use, as with other hypnotics, should be limited.

Although these factors may explain the huge preference of clinicians for the benzodiazepines, it is worth emphasizing that the patient's preference is of greater importance. One would be loath to change a patient from a drug which he has found to be acceptable and beneficial, even though it might not be one's ordinary first choice.

PRINCIPLES IN CLINICAL USE

Mies van der Rohe's famous dictum about architecture, "Less is more," applies to these drugs. Using them less may better use them. Unless physicians learn to use these drugs with restraint, political pressures steming from the growing problem of drug abuse may lead to unwise constraints.

Concomitant Non-Drug Treatments

First, anxiety is clearly related to life experiences. "Psychotherapy" and altering the environment may be more to the point. Use of drugs, at least in our present understanding, should be considered no more than symptomatic, adjunctive treatment. "Psychotherapy" has always been put into quotations in this review, simply because it has almost as many meanings as it has practitioners. Some purists have maintained that it is impossible to do effective psychotherapy in the presence of drug treatment, as the presence of anxiety is a motivating force for psychotherapy. Little proof exists for such an assertion. If anxiety can be so totally relieved by drug treatment as to make the patient unwilling to entertain another treatment, then perhaps the latter isn't really indicated.

No one has yet tried to exploit fully the interaction of metapharmacological influences and antianxiety drugs. From what we know already, it would seem reasonable to try to maximize the patient's belief in the treatment. On the other hand, some patients, who react to anxiety by extrovertive behavior and physical activity, tolerate sedative drugs poorly. Such patients often complain of being made more anxious by sedatives, and should be treated with smaller than usual doses, if at all.

Duration of Treatment

Anxiety is often episodic, waxing and waning with changes in one's life. In such cases, treatment might follow the course, drugs being used only when symptoms are discomforting or disabling and not indefinitely. Such episodes of treatment might be limited to a week. If anxiety is relieved, it might remain so without drugs. The knowledge that relief is available may sustain the patient over subsequent episodes. By limiting treatment to short courses, problems of tolerance with loss of efficacy, or increased doses with the risk of physical dependence, are avoided.

Not all patients who complain of anxiety have it episodically. Some have it chronically, and this may simply represent an unusually high level of "trait" anxiety. These patients often do very well with small doses of some antianxiety drug maintained indefinitely. Generally, one need not worry about physical dependence developing in such patients, although undoubtedly they have some degree of psychological dependence to the drug.

Doses and Dosage Schedules

Doses must be titrated against the patient's need for relief from symptoms and his ability to function without mental impairment. Patients vary widely in their requirements for these drugs. Plasma concentrations of meprobamate vary over a three-fold range in patients receiving the same dose. The patient's tolerance to the drug may be tested by giving the initial doses when he is at home in the evening hours; if he gets sleepy then, little harm is done.

In determining dose, one must also pay some attention to the drugs the patient takes socially. A person who is a coffee addict, taking several cups during the day, may actually be aggravating his anxiety by the use of this drug. Rather than increasing his consumption of an antianxiety drug, he might best be advised to change his habits. On the other hand, a patient who customarily consumes alcoholic beverages, either during the day or evening hours, should avoid concomitant use of antianxiety drugs at the time of drinking.

Traditional divided dosage schedules of the tid or qid type make little sense. Most of these drugs have rather long plasma half-lives, ranging from 12 to 30 hours, so that frequent doses are not required. Any patient so troubled by anxiety that drug treatment is required should also have trouble sleeping. By giving the major portion of the daytime dose of drug at night, one capitalizes on its hypnotic effect. The long half-life assures some daytime carryover of effects, which is precisely the type of mild sedation desired during daytime activities. *Ad hoc* doses of much smaller size may be used by the patient as his symptoms during the day may require. Many patients discover this dosage schedule for themselves and prefer it over the fixed, traditional schedules. Customary doses of antianxiety drugs are shown in Table 5-II.

COMBINATIONS OF DRUGS

The combination of antianxiety drugs with antipsychotics was covered in Chapter 2 and with antidepressants in Chapter 4.

Table 5-II

Dosage Guide for Antianxiety Drugs

Generic Names	*Total Daily Dosage in Mgs (Divided into 2-4 Doses)*
Barbiturates	
phenobarbital	32-100
butabarbital	45-120
Glycerol Derivatives	
meprobamate	800-3200
tybamate	750-3000
Benzodiazepine Derivatives	
chlordiazepoxide	15-300
diazepam	5-60
oxazepam	30-120
Diphenylmethane Antihistaminics	
hydroxyzine	75-400
diphenhydramine	50-200
Phenothiazine Antipsychotic	
trifluoperazine	2-10
Tricyclic Antidepressant	
doxepin	10-50

Antianxiety Drugs Combined With Each Other

Very little seems to be gained from such combinations. Their use in clinical practice is relatively uncommon compared to other overuses of drug combinations. As most of the sedative-hypnotic antianxiety drugs have similar pharmacological effects, little more can be gained by adding another drug that cannot be gained by simply increasing the dose of the single drug. It is quite possible that a combination might reduce rather than enhance efficacy. One might argue with somewhat more logic for combinations of sedative-hypnotic with sedative-autonomic antianxiety drugs, as in this instance the mechanisms of action may be different between the two groups. Yet as indicated in the discussion of combinations of antianxiety drugs with antipsychotics and antidepressants, very little advantage is gained.

Combinations With Other Types of Drugs

The time-honored combination of belladonna and barbiturate has been mimicked in a thousand ways by pharmaceutical companies looking for a new product. While the anticholinergic drugs are most commonly combined with antianxiety drugs (not only phenobarbital but also meprobamate and chlordiazepoxide), the list has been extended to others, such as estrogens, anorexics, analgesics and coronary vasodilators. The need for antianxiety drugs in many patients taking these other drugs may be minimal. When such combinations seem to be needed, they might best be determined extemporaneously, which generally allows much more flexibility of dose and dosage schedules.

SIDE EFFECTS AND COMPLICATIONS

Therapeutic Doses

One must always be concerned when prescribing sedative drugs lest they interfere with the performance of some dangerous activity, such as driving an automobile. Trading a mild degree of motor impairment for relief of anxiety may not be all bad, as disturbed emotional states must certainly contribute much to the dangers of driving. By titrating the dose of drug to the patient in the evening hours, and giving the major portion of it at bedtime, one should be able to get by with few and small doses during the day. These should be timed so as to avoid having their major impact at a time when driving must be done.

Although there has been a great deal of loose talk about "iatrogenic" drug abuse, the total amount of drug abuse of this sort is small compared with that which originates elsewhere. Patients may increase their doses of drugs without telling their doctors, and they may obtain multiple prescriptions to satisfy their needs, but these instances, while dramatic, are fairly infrequent. This does not relieve the physician of the responsibility for at least monitoring carefully the amount of drugs he prescribes and the frequency of prescriptions for any given patient. For a patient to be deprived of an effective therapy that would make his life more comfortable and fruitful because of some vague fear of drug abuse would be tragic. The relative safety of benzodiazepines and phenobarbital as drugs of abuse has been mentioned earlier, as well as some possible explanations for it. It is possible to induce withdrawal reactions from excessive doses of chlordiazepoxide or diazepam, but the symptoms appear gradually, the syndrome is attenuated over time, and withdrawal seizures, when they occur, are usually quite late, often as long as eight days after withdrawal (98). Thus, long-acting drugs seem to have some built-in safety mechanisms against producing severe withdrawal reactions. Although some patients may develop psychological dependence to these drugs, as they will to virtually all mind-altering drugs, instances of physical signs of dependence have been uncommon in clinical practice. Withdrawal reactions from meprobamate are severe, usually peaking within 12 to 48 hours after discontinuation of the drug (97). As some signs of physical dependence may be observed with only two to three times the usual therapeutic doses of this drug, many clinicians are loath to use meprobamate. Still, instances of abuse of this drug, either during medical treatment or as a "street drug" are relatively uncommon. The sedative-autonomic drugs are unlikely candidates for abuse as their autonomic side effects would make excessive doses intolerable.

Toxic Doses

The lack of fatal outcomes from overdoses of benzodiazepines is a great factor in explaining their popularity. The phenothiazines also share a high degree of safety in this regard, but for other reasons are not nearly so popular. All the other drugs mentioned as potential antianxiety drugs can be fatal if taken with suicidal intent.

Meprobamate has been fatal when taken in doses as small as 20 gm (fifty 400 mg tablets), though recoveries have occurred after doses of 40 gm. As sedatives are often taken in combination with other drugs or with alcohol, it is difficult to be certain about the contributing factors to mortality from overdoses of these drugs. The clinical picture of this intoxication resembles that of barbiturates and the management is the same. The relatively small amount of meprobamate excreted by the kidney as compared to the hepatic metabolism suggests that forced diuresis may be of limited value in these cases, but no doubt it should still be part of a generally supportive treatment program. Despite the popularity of this drug, it is still a relatively infrequent cause of suicide as compared with barbiturates. Perhaps the large size of the tablets acts as a deterrent. A chemical homolog, tybamate, has a very short biological half-life and should be free of suicidal potential.

It is probably impossible to commit suicide with chlordiazepoxide or diazepam. No deaths were encountered in 22 instances of overdosage of the former drug, even with doses of up to 2.25 gm (ninety 25 mg capsules). After observing 121 cases of poisoning with chlordiazepoxide in patients from 15 months to 63 years of age, the conclusion was reached that when the drug was used alone, symptoms were quite mild, consisting only of drowsiness or stupor. When the drug was used in combination with others, the effects of the second drug always predominated. Two instances of diazepam overdosage in children have been relatively mild. Toxic effects of overdosage are deep stupor and coma, marked muscle relaxation, but little fall in blood pressure or respiratory depression. Supportive treatment is usually enough. The new analogs, such as oxazepam, should prove to be equally innocuous and briefer in their effects. As anxious patients are often issued large supplies of drugs between visits to the physician, it is easy to order an amount which could be lethal. The availability of such safe and effective sedatives as drugs of this type is a definite advantage (106).

SUMMARY

Anxiety is a ubiquitous symptom which occurs in normal persons as well as those with severe physical or emotional disorders. Its manifestations and severity are related both to the character of the patient and to his life experiences. Difficulties in evaluating the efficacy of antianxiety drugs are many, but their widespread and growing medical use confirms their utility. The benzodiazepines, exemplified by chlordiazepoxide and diazepam, are the most popular agents, offering certain advantages over others. Meprobamate, phenobarbital, small doses of antipsychotics or certain tricyclic antidepressants, antihistaminics, and other drugs with sedative actions are also available and may be useful in selected patients. Antianxiety drugs interact with personality characteristics of the patient and with attitudes of the physician either to produce favorable or unfavorable responses. The decision to use these drugs should not deny patients other forms of treatment. Doses and dosage schedules should be tailored to the needs of individual patients, rather than following some rote pattern. Interrupted brief courses of treatment are feasible for many patients and may prevent overuse with possible tolerance and habituation. Fears of side effects, especially physical dependence, should not discourage their use when they are truly indicated.

CHAPTER 6

DRUGS IN CHILDREN

$\rm F$EW areas in the application of psychotherapeutic drugs are more uncertain and controversial than their use in children. To some extent, this is the result of much less interest than in the exploitation of these drugs in adults. As is the case elsewhere in clinical pharmacology, children are "therapeutic orphans." Not only does one have the problem of what constitutes "informed consent" in children, but also the fact that children with psychiatric disorders seldom present emergent indications for drug treatment which are present in those afflicted with medical disorders. Whatever one says about the use of psychotherapeutic drugs in children is likely to be contentious.

SPECIAL PROBLEMS

Diagnosis

A major problem in studying drugs for treating children is to establish an accurate diagnosis. Many diagnostic schemes have been proposed. In one, adolescent behavior disorders were fitted into four major categories: (a) behavior disturbances such as hyperactivity, delinquency, or sociopathic-aggressive behavior; (b) organic brain syndromes, such as epilepsies, brain damage from birth, trauma or disease, or so-called minimal brain damage with only borderline neurologic signs and EEG abnormalities; (c) schizophrenias of the usual types, in addition to childhood autism; and (d) affective disorders, chiefly depression, in postpubertal children. Many young patients do not fall into these categories, so that a purely empiric approach is necessary in some, using graded ratings of symptoms and signs. Such standardization of descriptive aspects of these disorders might be helpful in allaying the present confusion engendered by multiple, ill-defined diagnostic terms and subsequent therapeutic manipulations (66).

Another diagnostic classification was proposed by an international study group, involving three axes. The first revolved around the usual clinical psychiatric syndromes, such as normal variation; adaptation reaction; specific developmental disorder (the hyperkinetic child is an example); conduct disorder; neurotic disorder; psychosis (a schizophrenic child would be an example); personality disorder; "psychosomatic" disorder; other disorders (anorexia nervosa would be an example); and mental abnormality existing alone. A second axis revolved around intellectual functioning, with a range from normal to severe impairment. The third axis revolved around associated or presumed etiological factors, such as diseases of the various organ systems; malformation; developmental disorders; and various social or emotional environmental factors (199).

Obviously, there are many ways one can cut the diagnostic pie. One might wonder why it is worth cutting at all, except for the fact that considerable evidence from the use of drugs in adults suggests that results are best when an accurate diagnosis is made.

Smaller Changes in Clinical Manifestations

Children seldom show the dramatic changes shown by adults, such as the rapid resolution of symptoms of psychosis or depression often observed when adults receive proper drug treatment. This difference may signify that these disorders in children are intrinsically more severe. If one subscribes to the view that schizophrenia and endogenous depression have a strong genetic-biochemical basis, then, as is usually the case with other genetic disorders, the earlier the appearance of phenotypical manifestations, the more severe the genetic load. The most dramatic example is the case of childhood autism, which is so severe a disorder that many view it as distinct from schizophrenia. Yet it may be argued that with enough genetic load, any schizophrenic might show these manifestations, and indeed, some adult schizophrenics do.

Difficulties in Drug Evaluation

Children are developing organisms and some degree of change is always expected. The simple process of maturation may provide gains that cannot be attributed to treatments. A child, even more than an adult, is highly responsive to changes in environment, relations with others (particularly parents and siblings) and to the expectations of those treating him. While placebo controls may sometimes be omitted in evaluating drugs in adults, such is seldom the case in children. Finally, the sources of information about changes in children are less direct, being less likely to come from the patient and more likely from others who observe his behavior (61).

HYPERKINETIC OR MINIMALLY BRAIN DAMAGED CHILDREN

Diagnosis

The "hyperkinetic" or "minimal brain dysfunction" (MBD) child is characterized by poor attention span, distractability, emotional lability, aggressiveness, and hyperactivity. Sometimes the diagnosis is easy. The child is driven by an uncontrollable urge to move, purposelessly and continually. He races from one idea to another, without being able to sustain his attention. These two symptoms, increased activity and distractability, are the primary components. The diagnosis may be made a little more secure if the electroencephalogram (EEG) proves to be abnormal, although an abnormal EEG alone is not diagnostic. So-called "soft" neurological signs may also be present: mild visual or hearing impairments; crossed-eyes or fine, jerky, lateral eye movements; poor fine visual-motor coordination; confusion of laterality, with frequent left-handedness.

An attempt has been made to define diagnostic criteria (130). According to the scheme presented, the diagnosis should be made if seven of nine of the following signs and symptoms are present:

(1) hyperactivity; (2) low tolerance for frustration; (3) aggressive behavior; (4) impulsive behavior; (5) seeking companionship; (6) inability to postpone gratification, such as demanding behavior or lack of sustained effort; (7) poor school performance; (8) poor peer relationships; and (9) hostile and rebellious behavior. If more than two of the following five symptoms and signs of hypokinetic behavior are present, the diagnosis might be questioned: (1) depression; (2) sullen, seclusive behavior; (3) indifferent, passive behavior; (4) mood swings; (5) withdrawal.

The manifold symptoms of this vague disorder of children are nonspecific. They may also be symptoms or signs of a normal but neglected child; or a child with mental retardation, schizophrenia or depression; or a child with specific learning disabilities; or perhaps a child with frequent petit mal epileptic attacks. Obviously, such a confusing assortment of disorders may not be easily separated by casual observation. Diagnosing such disordered behavior in children can challenge the mettle of the most skilled child psychiatrist. Because the diagnosis of borderline cases is difficult, some children are probably undiagnosed, while others may be diagnosed inappropriately. Sometimes the diagnosis is established on the basis of a therapeutic trial with stimulant drugs.

The school teacher may be the first to recognize symptoms and signs of learning disability and poor social behavior. Parents are often loath to see any abnormality in their children, a natural reaction. Even when it is recognized, they hope that as the child goes to school he will "grow" out of it. So it may become the teacher's unpleasant, but helpful, job to raise the issue of diagnostic referral.

Prevalence

The MBD syndrome is found in about three of every one hundred school children in the United States. Estimates vary between geographic areas an socioeconomic groups, being higher in urban poor than in suburban middleclass children. Boys are affected several times as often as girls, for reasons not clear. The disorder is worldwide, although some countries claim to have an exceedingly low prevalence. Its suspected cause is implicit in its name. A degree of brain dysfunction, based either on genetic or environmental conditions, is assumed; some would aver that it is often far from "minimal." Among environmental causes might be illnesses or infections in the mother during pregnancy, a difficult labor, or some infection or injury early in life. Yet for many of these children, psychological or social factors may be more evident than biological causes.

Prognosis

Although some children seem to undergo a spontaneous remission at about age 12, especially if they have been adequately treated, those children who are untreated have a much higher risk of later becoming delinquent, schizophrenic, or having some other psychiatric disorder (229). Thus, proper recognition of the disorder and its early treatment are highly desirable.

Stimulant Drugs

In 1937 it was observed that some "hyperkinetic" children improved remarkably when treated with amphetamine (21). This observation has been repeatedly confirmed over the past 35 years. Such a result has been considered to be "paradoxical," for one would expect a stimulant drug to make matters worse rather than better. It is still uncertain how these drugs provide their benefits, or in which children. An interesting observation is that children who respond less to stimuli during psychophysiological testing respond best to stimulants. Thus the afflicted child is actually underaroused, the drugs acting in their expected fashion rather than paradoxically. Another idea is that MBD children can't screen out useless or irrelevant sensory information; the drugs activate an inhibitory pathway in the brain which monitors sensory input better (38). Here, too, the drugs would not be acting paradoxically. In general, best results from stimulant drug therapy are obtained in children who show the most "organicity," that is, who have a history of some abnormality during pregnancy, birth or infancy, or who show some of the soft neurological signs and EEG abnormalities previously mentioned (134).

Since 1937, sympathomimetic stimulants have remained the drugs of choice over more recently introduced sedatives or antipsychotics (39). The preferred stimulant drug has become methylphenidate, largely because of unjustified fears that use of dextroamphetamine may predispose to its later abuse; no such sequence has been documented. The customary doses of dextroamphetamine range between 10 and 30 mg daily, with those of methylphenidate being approximately double. Doses are usually divided. Some patients seem to require more frequent dosage than others to avoid brief periods of emotional lability as the effect of the drug wears off. In such cases, it might make sense to attempt to prolong the span of action of dextroamphetamine by administering a dose of sodium bicarbonate to alkalinize the urine and decrease its rate of excretion. Fortunately, any beneficial effects from stimulant drugs are usually evident fairly soon, usually within the first three weeks of treatment. Courses of treatment are often geared to the school year, with vacation periods being used for testing possible withdrawal of drug. The drug program may be resumed only if relapse occurs.

Sometimes response to drugs can be used as a diagnostic test. If the response is favorable, and this will usually be quickly apparent, then one assumes that the diagnosis is correct. Children who respond best to dextroamphetamine seem to have an unusual tolerance for the drug, possibly related to a more rapid excretion (59). Failure to respond occurs in one-third to one-half of MBD children. This high failure rate may be due to misdiagnosis, to inadequate use of the drugs, or to the fact that the syndrome may have multiple causes. After all, our behavioral repertoire is fairly limited and the same symptom, restlessness, may be seen in a wide variety of emotional and neurological disorders. Some children who fail to respond to stimulants may later respond to other drugs, such as tranquilizers and antidepressants, which might imply misdiagnosis.

One is not anxious to embark on treatment with drugs in children if they can be avoided. The most enthusiastic proponents of drug treatment are the parents of children who have a good response. Consequently, it would be tragic to miss the opportunity to help a child because of some prejudice against drug treatment.

Are the stimulants likely to have unwanted effects? Yes, all drugs do. These are most likely to be sleeplessness and diminished appetite, although these two major side effects of stimulant drugs are usually infrequent in MBD children. Is there a risk of making the child dependent on stimulant drugs later on? The current widespread use of stimulants by adolescents makes this a reasonable concern. Evidence from thirty-five years of use of these drugs says "no." It should be remembered that these drugs do not create a "high" in MBD children.

Concomitant Treatment

The most ardent advocate of drug therapy would not view this treatment either as the sole of major treatment of these children. Special classes and teaching techniques are imperative for these children; to rely on drugs rather than proper teaching is reprehensible. Perceptual-motor training should be part of such special programs. Some children may also require psychotherapy for some of the secondary effects of their disorder, such as the poor relationships with classmates, siblings or parents. As school teachers may have the greatest opportunity to observe the MBD child during a variety of social and learning experiences, school personnel should be included in the treatment program. They are uniquely able to provide the valuable feedback necessary to evaluate treatment.

SCHIZOPHRENIA

Schizophrenia in children can be a disaster, for the afflicted individual for his parents and for his siblings. As increasing evidence suggests that schizophrenia is a genetic disorder, its appearance in early childhood may be construed as evidence of a more severe disorder with a less favorable course than that of adult-onset schizophrenia. One of the cruelest conceptions in psychiatry is that which blames the parents, specifically the mother, for a child's schizophrenic illness. It is truly an instance of adding insult to injury.

Types of Childhood Schizophrenia

Several types of schizophrenia in childhood have been described. Many of the symptoms are the same as those seen in adult disorder: (1) lack of firm self-identity; (2) fantastic thinking, behavior and feelings; (3) both impaired and precocious, or spotty, psychological functioning; (4) loss of normal interests, or the appearance of unusual or regressive ones; (5) disturbances of language, either in amount attained, or in content, rhythm, intonation, pitch, stress or volume; (6) deficient social relationships with a tendency towards social withdrawal. Specific types include:

(a) *Early infantile autism* — This disorder appears in infancy and is characterized by self-isolation; fear of novelty; language delay or distortion; repetitive movements, often whirling; and disparate abilities. The children may seem to be insensitive in pain, biting themselves or butting their head against the wall. They lack normal eye contact and give a feeling of total detachment. They resist change and meticulously repeat behaviors. Sometimes they may excel in some special ability, such as drawing or memorizing, while functioning at a retarded level in most other psychological functions. Indeed, the diagnosis may be confused with severe mental retardation.

(b) *Symbiotic infantile psychosis* — This form of the disorder appears between two and four years of age after an apparent normal early development. It is characterized by many of the same symptoms noted above, as well as an inability to separate the child's self-image from that of his mother or her surrogates.

(c) *Pseudoneurotic schizophrenia* — This disorder appears even later, usually during the school years. At first the symptoms may suggest a neurosis, with anxiety, phobias and obsessive-compulsive symptoms predominating. Later, some of the more definite characteristics of schizophrenia appear, such as repetitive questioning, bizarre rituals and mannerisms. There may be shifts between neurotic and psychotic behavior.

(d) *Pseudopsychopathic schizophrenia* — The onset of this form of illness is insidious during adolescence and is most often manifested by some delinquent, impulsive, acting-out behavior.

Patients may retain some insight and effectively cover their psychotic thinking, but eventually the more characteristic clinical manifestations of schizophrenia appear (3).

Drug Therapy

Drug therapy of schizophrenic children has generally been less successful than it has been in treating the adult disorder. Not only may this reflect the greater severity of the disorder in children, but it may also result from a diminished capacity for social learning at a crucial stage in life. Because of the uncertain and sometimes disappointing results of drug therapy, some clinicians are inclined to try almost anything else first. This point of view has little justification for, as with adult schizophrenia, traditional psychotherapeutic measures have a barely discernible effect. Rather, one should use drugs as needed and try to exploit whatever benefit they may produce to provide the handicapped child the learning and social skills that anyone must have to reach their fullest potential.

Almost all the known antipsychotic drugs have been used with some degree of benefit in schizophrenic children. As with adults, it is often difficult to predict in advance which drug may produce the best possible result. The choice of drug may be based on the agitated-withdrawn continuum, using sedative phenothiazines, such as chlorpromazine and thioridazine in agitated children, and more specific antipsychotics, such as trifluoperazine in withdrawn children (60). Neither is there any evidence to suggest that any single antipsychotic drug is preferable to another in terms of efficacy.

Children, as well as young adults, are especially vulnerable to the acute dystonic reactions produced by most antipsychotic drugs. Often these occur at less than optimal antipsychotic doses of drug, so that concurrent treatment with some anticholinergic drug may be required. Elixir of diphenhydramine is especially useful, not only in preventing this complication, but also in providing some additional sedative action. The relative lack of this neurological complication with thioridazine may make this drug preferable in some respects, although sedation may interfere with other rehabilitative measures.

One usually starts with low doses of drug, gradually increasing doses until such time as side effects limit further increases (at least without other treatment being added) or until therapeutic effects are attained. Divided doses are preferable during this early stage of dose-ranging, but later on one may wish to diminish daytime doses and give the major dose at night. Probably more often than in adults one would like to try interrupted courses of treatment. The first reason for doing this is to ascertain that the drug is really having a beneficial effect, something that may be difficult to appreciate until the child begins to relapse to his initial state. Another reason for doing so is to try to reduce the possibility of late-appearing dyskinesias or some other long-term complication of drug therapy. Finally, evidence suggests that chlorpromazine, and quite possibly other antipsychotic drugs, interferes with release of growth hormone. Interrupted courses may avoid a permanent alteration in the child's predicted growth pattern.

It is quite realistic to view the schizophrenic child as one might any child handicapped by some sensory defect, such as poor vision and deafness, or some musculoskeletal disorder, such as paralysis or loss of a limb. One wants to exploit all his possible advantages so as to train him to overcome the handicap. Thus, social, educational and vocational programs must be geared to a realistic life adjustment rather than striving to attain what for many children is an unattainable normal degree of function. These ancillary services are a must for such handicapped children, for without them, no child can be considered as to have been adequately treated. Even with them, results are too often disappointing in terms of any productive life adjustment. Unless there is some reason to believe that the family environment is detrimental to the child, or vice versa, schizophrenic children are far better off in their own homes than in institutions. Lacking an adequate natural family, placement in an understanding, benevolent and well-indoctrinated foster family can be quite helpful.

DEPRESSION

Depressions are commonly thought to be limited to the middle and later epochs of life. The rather high, and increasing, rate of suicide among adolescents is clear evidence that depression may also occur early in life. If one believes in a genetic biochemical basis for endogenous depression, then one might assume that with a strong enough genetic load, such depression could occur at any time of life. Naturally, the life situation of the child plays an important role. It is possible to induce depression in almost any infant purely by psychological measures, namely the separation of the child from its mother or a mother surrogate.

Characteristics of Childhood Depression

Symptoms of depression in children may mislead. They are often physical, rather than clear disturbances of mood or behavior. Nonspecific recurrent abdominal pain, headache, sleep difficulties, irrational fears, irritability, unaccountable tearfulness and temper outbursts may represent some of the unusual symptoms of depression in children. Behavioral changes may provide a clue, such as social withdrawal, aggressive or antisocial behavior, and school failure. Most depressed children have a strong family history of depression in about one-third of close relatives (69). Such a relationship does not really settle the question of nature versus nurture, however, for a depressed parent might transmit this mood to his child by psychological rather than genetic influences.

Drug Treatment of Childhood Depression

As is the case with depression in adults, not all useful drugs are limited to those usually termed "antidepressant." Good results have been attained with other types of drugs, such as chlordiazepoxide and phenothiazines. The MAO inhibitor, phenelzine, has been reputed to be fairly effective in children, but in view of less dramatic results in adults, as well as its considerable dangers, should not be viewed as a treatment of first choice. Imipramine or some other tricyclic drug should be tried first, especially if the child shows symptoms reminiscent of the adult retarded depression, such as social withdrawal and lessened motor movements. As many of the depressive syndromes in children more often resemble the anxious depressions of adult life, these may best respond to chlordiazepoxide or other antianxiety drugs. The latter in children include the sedative antihistaminics, such as hydroxyzine. Phenelzine, in combination with an antianxiety drug such as chlordiazepoxide, may be effective in phobias associated with childhood depression, just as it is in phobic states in adults. Because of the atypical manifestations of depression in children, clear distinctions between depressive subtypes are not easy, so that choice of drug may have to be more or less empiric.

Imipramine and amitriptyline have been found to be useful in preventing enuresis in children, even in the absence of clear evidence of an associated depression. The mode of action may be by altering sleep patterns so that the loss of control characteristic of enuresis does not occur.

MENTAL DEFICIENCY

The great hope for a drug which increases mental capacity has not yet been realized. Drugs currently available can only influence the mentally retarded by indirect actions, such as controlling motor behavior and distractability, which in turn may lead to increased attention span and better intellectual performance. Treatment is entirely symptomatic and any gains are likely to be small ones.

The earliest reports of the effects of reserpine and chlorpromazine in treating mentally retarded children and adults were quite glowing: behavior was controlled, self-care markedly increased and intelligence quotients raised. The more sober view of recent years is that while most of these changes may occur, their degree is far less than originally thought, and a sizable number of patients obtain none of these benefits.

Virtually all antipsychotic drugs have now been tried in mentally defective children and adults with similar small gains. Their most important use is in controlling motor agitation, which may be remarkable persistent and severe in such patients. Thioridazine is often preferred because of its comparatively greater sedative effects and a lesser propensity to evoke dystonic reactions or the Parkinson syndrome (5). Dextroamphetamine usually makes these patients worse, again suggesting that it really does not work paradoxically in children. If drugs likely to evoke severe extrapyramidal reactions are used, such as haloperidol, one might be well advised to use some anti-Parkinson drug prophylactically, so that effective doses can be used (47). That the beneficial effects of these drugs may be due to nonspecific sedation rather than their specific antipsychotic action is indicated by a study which found no difference between nortriptyline (which is sedative), pentobarbital sodium and chlorpromazine, all of which were superior to placebo (29). Despite large doses of these drugs, severely retarded children may not have their hyperactivity controlled. One cannot help wondering if augmentation of treatment with lithium would be beneficial.

GENERAL PRINCIPLES IN USING PSYCHOTHERAPEUTIC DRUGS IN CHILDREN

Despite the fact that pediatric psychopharmacology has fallen far behind the study of drugs in adults, perhaps it is just as well. Children are not ideal candidates on which to evaluate brand new drugs. It turns out that in many respects, the principles which apply to the use of drugs in adults apply equally to children (57, 230).

Here are some notions for which there is reasonable consensus:

1. Drugs may be quite useful in children, but establishing a correct diagnosis and selection of the best possible drug is paramount, as it is with most other types of drug therapy.

2. The better one knows the pharmacological effects of the drugs, the better one can anticipate their side effects, which are most often extensions of their pharmacological effects. Warning about possible side effects is especially important when treating children, lest both parent and child become so alarmed by them that they will no longer consider drug treatment.

3. Drugs should not be used for trivial indications in children, especially not a a sop to parents. One should be convinced that the situation is not due to some self-limited condition, that the problem is serious enough to justify all the risks of drug therapy, and that one can provide the proper clinical controls and

precautions to avoid serious complications.

4. Familiar drugs are generally preferred over the newer ones, at least until the latter have had fairly extensive trials in adults.

5. Doses are flexible and variable; there is no fixed therapeutic dose. Dosage schedules should be geared to fit the pharmacokinetics of the drug.

6. Interrupted treatment may be used in lieu of placebo control to determine that the drug is really efficacious, that it is still required, and to reduce the possibility of tolerance or some complication due to cumulative doses.

7. Drugs in children, even more than in adults, require other concomitant treatments or services if best results are to be obtained.

8. Drugs should not be used in acute stress or adjustment reactions where the cause is clearly apparent, such as a change in home or school, an illness, or separation from a friend. These episodes are usually self-limiting and it might be best for the child's future development to work through them psychologically rather than to seek help from a bottle.

SUMMARY

Children with psychiatric disorders present special problems in the use of psychotherapeutic drugs. Accurate diagnoses are more difficult to make and responses to treatment less easily evaluated. Hyperkinetic or minimally brain damaged children may respond specifically to stimulant drugs. As these symptoms may be confounded with those of other childhood disorders, misdiagnosis may occur and other types of drugs be found to be effective. Schizophrenia and depression in childhood may represent more serious forms of the disorder than those which appear in adult life. The indications and principles of use for antipsychotic and antidepressant drugs are somewhat similar in children to those which should be followed in using these drugs in adults. Results from drug therapy of childhood psychiatric disorders are less dramatic than in adults, and far more than in the latter; drug therapy should be accompanied by rigorous social, educational and vocational rehabilitative measures. Treatment of mental deficiency with drugs aims only at the control of disturbing symptoms; no drug remedies the primary defect. Despite a prevailing conservative approach to drug treatment in children with psychiatric disorders, much benefit may be obtained from their appropriate use.

CHAPTER 7

MISCELLANEOUS DISORDERS

PSYCHOSES ASSOCIATED WITH OLD AGE

THESE disorders would include principally pre--
senile, senile, arteriosclerotic and mixed types of brain syndromes.
Ordinarily psychoses of old age begin insidiously and progress
gradually. Sometimes a tenuous balance may be easily upset, and
some severe medical illness or difficult surgical procedure may
produce a decompensation that is irreversible. Acute changes which
resemble those of senile psychoses may be the first herald of some
serious and sometimes remediable medical illness, such as congestive
heart failure, occult malignancy, or brain tumor. Many older people,
especially those who live alone, who are edentulous, or who are
poor, suffer from under-nutrition. This alone, or particularly if
complicated by alcohol ingestion, may mimic the mental changes of
senility. Besides alcohol, other drugs may be at fault. Older persons
are especially vulnerable to the deliriant properties of many
anticholinergic drugs which may be used to treat depression,
Parkinson's disease, or diverticulitis. Even schizophrenia may make
its first appearance in old age. Thus, these diagnoses should not be a
wastebasket in which to categorize all mental disturbances of old
age, but rather a challenge to one's general medical acumen. The
effort is worthwhile, for in some instances a still productive life may
be saved.

Other Pathogenetic Considerations

A metabolic disorder for senile psychoses is suggested by the
spotty neurofibrillary degeneration and senile plaque formation,
but whatever it may be is unknown. The multiple areas of small
cerebral infarcts, which may make brain sections resemble a swiss
cheese, are associated with local vascular occlusion or thrombosis.
In either case, the damage to the nervous system is irreversibly.
Treatment, no matter how specific it might be, would more likely

prevent future rather than repair past damage.

The fact that some "senile" patients show improvement following improved social care has weakened the correlation between brain damage and the level of impairment. Obviously, poverty, isolation and physical illness may impair the mental capacity of the aged and mimic the senile state. When these causes are excluded, however, it is generally agreed that the degree of impairment correlates positively with the degree of pathology.

Drug Treatment

Treatment has been aimed at postulated specific causes; general nutritional (vitamins, amino acid supplements, digestive enzymes, anabolic steroids), specific nutrients (glutamic acid, yeast ribonucleic acid, adenosine-5-monophosphate), circulatory disorders (niacin, nicotinic acid alcohol, cyclandelate, hydrogenated ergot alkaloids), or arteriosclerosis (heparin and other anticoagulants, thyroxine analogs, vegetable oils and other lipid-lowering agents). No specific proof of the efficacy of any of these postulated mechanisms is valid, with the exception of impaired circulation in the case of cerebral arteriosclerosis.

Analeptic-stimulant therapy with pentylenetetrazole still has its proponents, but almost all adequately controlled studies have been negative. Sympathomimetic stimulants may be dangerous or even aggravate irritability or psychotic symptoms. Tricyclic antidepressants may be used, but with great caution, in such patients who have a concurrent retarded depression. The peripheral and central anticholinergic actions of these drugs may cause severe side effects, including aggravation of the confused mental state. In addition hypotension has resulted in physical injuries due to falls, or possibly has precipitated myocardial infarctions.

Most symptomatic control of the psychosis of the aged has come from the judicious use of phenothiazines, such as acetophenazine or thioridazine. Irritability, disturbed sleep and careless personal hygiene may be alleviated. As in the case with tricyclic antidepressants, doses must be very low initially and adjusted with great care. The well-known propensity for paradoxical reactions to conventional sedatives in the elderly with agitation often being precipitated by drugs such as phenobarbital should be considered if the use of such drugs is contemplated. Until the basic mechanisms of these disorders are better understood, treatment will be limited to a purely symptomatic approach.

Lately, renewed interest in hydrogenated ergot alkaloids has appeared, despite earlier studies that indicated little utility. As these are alpha-adrenergic blocking drugs, they might be anticipated to dilate vessels constricted by noradrenergic influences. Evidence suggests that small vessels of the brain are under this control, just as are most peripheral arterioles. Whether augmented blood flow in the microcirculation of the brain can improve function must still be considered questionable (13). If this should prove to be the case, the beneficial effects of phenothiazines might also be attributed in part to this mechanism.

ALCOHOLISM

Despite the renewed concern about drugs of abuse, alcohol remains the most widely abused of all. The enormous morbidity and mortality associated with alcohol abuse make it a major contemporary public health problem.

We know relatively little about the pharmacological effects requisite for a drug of abuse, with the possible exception that the drug usually produces a pleasurable sensation in those who take it and that tolerance tends to develop. Although recent evidence suggests that alkaloids such as tetrahydropapaveroline may be formed from endogenous catecholamines in the presence of alcohol, there is little clinical or pharmacological evidence to indicate a common mechanism for alcohol and opiate abuse (53, 207). In addition, we do not know much about the psychological and social factors which enter into the choice of the drug of abuse.

Acute Alcoholism

Practicing physicians are frequently confronted with the treatment of acute alcoholics. Plasma concentrations of alcohol over 300 mg per 100 ml, especially if these are accompanied by other drugs or by unsuspected illnesses or injuries, may be rapidly fatal. Drugs may be required for control of disturbed behavior, but sedatives must be used carefully in the presence of high levels of blood alcohol lest unexpected fatalities occur. Supportive treatment often suffices, and when toxic levels of alcohol have been taken, dialysis by any technique may be life-saving by rapidly removing alcohol from the body. Attempts to hasten the metabolism of alcohol, which is a fixed, zero-order process, have generally been unsuccessful. Whether or not intravenous fructose will be helpful remains to be seen (144).

Chronic Alcoholism

Many alcoholics, especially after reaching some crisis in their lives or after a bout of delirium tremens, become dry for a while. The odds are overwhelming that they will once again resume drinking. Many types of interval treatment have been proposed. Aversive therapy, either with disulfiram or calcium carbimide, has only limited application. The coupling of the unpleasant interaction produced by these inhibitors of aldehyde dehydrogenase and alcohol may serve both as a deconditioning device as well as a direct deterrent (145). As the success of this program depends on the continued daily use of the aversive drug, an alcoholic may safely resume drinking within a couple of days of voluntary discontinuation of the treatment. Another possible aversive drug, metronidazole, has not lived up to its earlier promise (123).

Based on the notion that the compulsion to drink is due to a mounting level of anxiety, a number of antianxiety drugs have been substituted for alcohol with varying degrees of success. The early enthusiasm for antianxiety agents, such as chlordiazepoxide, as such treatments has been tempered by the fact that it is relatively easy to convert an addict from one drug to another. The ability of alcohol to induce enzymes for metabolizing drugs is well-known, and explains the enormous tolerance for common sedatives that many alcoholics develop. On the other hand, when high levels of blood alcohol prevail, the metabolizing enzymes are poisoned (198). Doses of sedatives which are ordinarily well tolerated may, when combined with the depressant effects of alcohol itself, become lethal. The number of unwitting suicides due to combinations of secobarbital sodium and alcohol continues to arise at an alarming rate.

Withdrawal Reactions to Alcohol

Alcohol withdrawal syndromes vary from the "shakes" to hyperthermic, and possibly fatal, delirium tremens (See Table 7-I). As the term implies, these syndromes appear in the presence of a declining or absent level of plasma alcohol. Consequently, many anonymous alcoholics become manifest only when some inter-current injury puts them into a hospital and removes the source of their drug. There are two major principles of treatment: (a) Replacement of alcohol with pharmacologically or physiologically equivalent drug, and (b) gradual withdrawal of the equivalent drug. For many years, drugs such as pentobarbital sodium, paraldehyde and chloral hydrate have been standard agents for substitution, but sedatives which may be somewhat safer in regard to respiratory depressant effects, such as chlordiazepoxide or chlormethiazole, have been recently introduced (120). So have other new drugs such as promazine, chlorpromazine, or hydroxyzine. The latter drugs are not the physiological equivalents required and are considerably less efficacious than those which are. Further, by lowering seizure threshold, they may aggravate the normal tendency towards withdrawal seizures.

The goal of treatment is to keep the patient in a state of light sleep until symptoms are controlled and gradual withdrawal of drug can be undertaken. Obviously, doses of substitutive drugs must be entirely flexible to meet the varying needs of patient. Exceedingly large doses, at least by usual standards, may be

Table 7-I

Alcohol-Barbiturate Abstinence Syndrome

Apprehension; muscle weakness on exertion; coarse, voluntary tremors; faintness; loss of appetite or vomiting; twitches or uncontrolled movements – 1st day; may last 3 to 14 days.

Epileptic seizures – 2nd or 3rd day; may last 8 days.

Psychosis, visual hallucinations, delirium – 3rd to 8th day; may last 3 to 14 days.

required; for example, doses of chlordiazopoxide of 600 to 800 mg daily are frequently necessary. Weaning from drug should be gradual and guided by the patient's clinical state. Most patients can be brought down to somewhat conventional sedative doses within a week.

The greatest value of drug therapy of milder alcohol withdrawal syndromes may be the prevention of more serious complications, such as frank delirium tremens or convulsions in a relatively few patients (127). Even frank delirium tremens has a favorable outcome if one provides good supportive treatment. No differential effect in delirium tremens was found between chlordiazepoxide, paraldehyde, perphenazine and pentobarbital sodium, although the first two were slightly preferable (121). Thus, drug treatment is not primary in alcoholic withdrawal states. Excellent medical supervision, with an alert eye for potentially dangerous medical and surgical complications, as well as good supportive treatment, is essential.

ABUSE OF SEDATIVE-HYPNOTIC DRUGS

Sedative-hypnotic drugs have been used medically for over seventy years. They have been used nonmedically for their intoxicating effects, which some individuals find to be pleasant, almost as long. During the past year, especially, nonmedical use of sedative-hypnotics by young persons has soared. It remains to be seen whether sedative-hypnotics are simply the "drug-of-the-year" or whether this increased use will persist. Fortunately, the new patterns of use are not much different from the old, so we know what to expect, even though we may be uncertain how to prevent it.

The belated proof, after almost 50 years of clinical use, of physical dependence from over-use of these drugs, led to a search for substitutes. In the 1950's, a number of barbiturate surrogates, such as glutethimide, or higher alcohols, such as ethchlorvynol, were introduced as hypnotics. Some quickly enjoyed wide use without evidence of greater efficacy or safety as compared with the barbiturates. Meprobamate was the first of a number of sedative or tranquilizer drugs designed to replace phenobarbital.

While meprobamate offered questionable advantages over phenobarbital, the benzodiazepines, exemplified by chlordiazepoxide and diazepam, were improvements. They were not necessarily more efficacious, although prevailing opinion is that they are, but they were far safer in regard to physical dependence and suicidal overdose. As many of these drugs are used as psychotherapeutic agents, their abuse potential should be considered.

Pharmacological Considerations of Abuse

Three pharmacological properties are shared by almost all drugs which present serious problems of abuse: tolerance, habituation, and physical dependence. These properties as they relate to sedative-hypnotic-antianxiety drugs will not be considered:

1. *Tolerance* – This term implies that increasing amounts of drug are required to maintain equal pharmacological effects. Tolerance is almost a requisite for development of physical dependence. Several types of tolerance are recognized. Metabolic tolerance signifies an increased ability of the body to dispose of the drug during continuing exposure to it. Phenobarbital is one of the most powerful inducers of drug-metabolizing enzymes known, increasing its own metabolism as well as that of many other drugs. Meprobamate shares this property, especially increasing its own metabolism, so that tolerance quickly develops. The benzodiazepines also stimulate drug-metabolizing enzymes, but less so than the other two types of drugs. Pharmacodynamic tolerance indicates a change in the sensitivity or numbers of receptors or cellular membrane macromolecules, upon which the drug acts. It may also include alterations in intracellular responses such as the rate of synthesis or release of neurohormones. Finally, psychic or behavioral tolerance may develop, persons using these drugs being able to compensate for certain deficits in function while maintaining other desired effects.

2. *Habituation* – This term is related somewhat to tolerance and is a requisite for physical dependence, yet it is separate from either. It signifies some reward to the user in terms of euphoria, greater confidence, or less depression, so that he is impelled to

continue its use without interruption. Not all drugs which are habituating are associated with tolerance or physical dependence. Marihuana, for instance, is habituating, but in man shows little evidence of tolerance or physical dependence.

3. *Physical dependence* — This term refers to a time-related syndrome which develops when a subject who has been overusing a drug suddenly stops taking it or sharply reduces its dose. Physical dependence on sedative-hypnotic drugs resembles that from alcohol, so that withdrawal reactions are called "alcohol-barbiturate" types. They consist of alterations of consciousness (delirium), neuromuscular irritability (tremors and seizures) and vegetative disturbances (vomiting, sweating, tachycardia). The syndrome of delirium tremens is well known. Recently it has been appreciated that the type of physical withdrawal reaction may be related to the plasma half-life of the drug. A drug with a very short half-life of six hours, such as the meprobamate homolog, tybamate, may never accumulate enough to create a consistently high tissue level. Drugs with very long half-lives or other active metabolites, such as chlordiazepoxide and most of the other benzodiazepines, have plasma half-lives of 36 to 48 hours after chronic administration. Thus, they contain some protection against the rapid fall in tissue levels of drug which provokes withdrawal reactions. Withdrawal reactions from these drugs are often subtle, mild and attenuated over time (98). Phenobarbital, besides having a long plasma half-life, is also slowly absorbed. Drugs with plasma half-lives in the range of 12 to 24 hours cause the most serious withdrawal reactions. These include meprobamate, and secobarbital, pentobarbital, or amobarbital sodium among the barbiturates. Ethanol, which has a relatively short plasma half-life, may produce some of its effects through other metabolites, possibly acetaldehyde

Abuse of Sedatives

Secobarbital sodium is the most popular sedative-hypnotic for abuse. The drug is rapidly absorbed, has a relatively short span of action (allowing for repeated surges of effects with repeated doses), is readily available and is relatively cheap. Methaqualone, a drug with history of abuse before being introduced into this country, is a current favorite for much the same reasons. Long-acting drugs do not provide the repeated surges of effect. Even though phenobarbital is as available and cheap as secobarbital sodium, its slow absorption and long action make it less desirable. The same situation prevails with benzodiazepines. In addition, the latter drugs are still under patent and come from a single source, so thaty are both much more expensive and much more carefully controlled than the generic drugs.

Strong suggestions have been made that medical use of these drugs may be related in an indirect but causative fashion to their nonmedical use. For instance, the children of parents who use alcohol or sedatives, either prescribed or purchased over-the-counter, are more likely to be drug users than those who are not. At first sight, such a relationship might imply that simply reducing the prescribing of these drugs for parents, or the promotion of over-the-counter remedies for nervousness might have a salutary effect. The situation may not be that simple. What this relationship may show is simply that children of parents who have high levels of psychopathology (if one wishes to view alcohol use as a manifestation of this) or who are more anxious or depressed than other parents (if we consider use of sedative-hypnotic drugs as a form of treatment for these disorders) are more likely than not to emulate their parents, either on a genetically or culturally-determined basis. Studies of patterns of use of prescribed sedative-hypnotic drugs show that their use is highest in those individuals who lack either strong family or religious ties. These same characteristics are found among the highest users of drugs among juveniles. Thus, the question of a relationship between medical and non-medical use of these drugs may be a complex one, even though in our desperation to do something constructive a simplistic interpretation is the most palatable one.

Withdrawal Reactions to Sedatives

Dependence on barbiturates and alcohol is so similar it is usually called "dependence of the alcohol-barbiturate" type. Treatment of withdrawal reactions to sedatives is based on the same general principles as that for alcohol withdrawal. When the sedative being used is short-acting, such as meprobamate or secobarbital sodium, one substitutes a longer-acting drug, such as pentobarbital sodium or phenobarbital. If an intrinsically long-acting drug has been abused, which is far less commonly the case, one might simply stay with that drug, but taper doses according to the usual schedules (See Table 7-II).

Treatment of Abuse of Sedatives

No such clear principles as those cited above guide the treatment of those who use sedatives in a spree fashion, or who do not reach the stage of physical dependence. Quite possibly, treatment might be best modelled after programs used for helping alcoholics, which might range over a wide variety of social-psychological techniques from the quasireligious aspects of Alcoholics Anonymous to more orthodox group therapy or therapeutic communities. Such an easy translation of techniques of managing alcoholics to sedative abusers may not be entirely realistic: The alcoholic usually uses only one, or at the most two, drugs, while abuse of sedatives may involve multiple drugs. Further, the alcoholic usually tries to exist within the prevailing cultural pattern; today's sedative abuser often spurns the prevailing culture for one that extolls drug use. Finally, the alcoholic may have more severe health problems and be older than the

Table 7-II

Principles in Managing Withdrawal Reactions
From Sedative-Hypnotics and Alcohol

General

1. Substitute equivalent drug
2. Gradually reduce dose

Specific

1. For secobarbital of meprobamate:
   pentobarbital, phenobarbital
2. For alcohol:
   pentobarbital, chloral hydrate, paraldehyde, chlordiazepoxide
3. For chlordiazepoxide or diazepam:
   continue same drugs in declining doses

relatively new and young breed of sedative users: He may be far more impelled to seek and accept treatment than the healthy novice.

On the more hopeful side, one would judge that abuse of sedative-hypnotic drugs may not lead to the long-lasting changes in bodily functions that make those who have abused alcohol or heroin forever vulnerable to any further use. This may simply be a difference between the pharmacodynamic effects of the different drugs or be due to the relatively shorter period of use that currently prevails with this class of drugs. Thus, rehabilitation by any means might be more long-lasting with the youthful users of sedative-hypnotic drugs than among those who abuse other drugs.

ABUSE OF OPIATES

Opiate abuse is currently epidemic in the United States and is showing an ominous increase in other countries of the Western World. Most of the abuse stems from "street" use. Despite the fact that millions of doses of opiates are given daily for medical purposes, documented cases of addiction from medical use of the drugs are rare. The abuse of these drugs is a complicated social phenomenon with many possible causes. Pharmacologically, opiates possess the major attributes of drugs of dependence, tolerance, habituation, and physical dependence. The most widely used drug is diacetylmorphine (heroin), almost exclusively of illicit manufacture. Other opiates or opioids are abused to a much lesser extent, and usually create less severe problems (44).

Withdrawal Reactions to Opiates

The principles in treating withdrawal reactions to opiates are essentially similar to those used for alcohol withdrawal, the substitution of a physiologically equivalent drug followed by gradual weaning. Methadone is the preferred agent for such substitution, the dose being based on the estimated daily intake of the primary addicting drug. Often the latter is estimated more in terms of money or "bags" than in milligrams, so that one must ordinarily rely heavily on the presence of symptoms and signs of withdrawal as the guide to dosage. Symptoms tend to be greatly exaggerated, so that objective manifestations, such as gooseflesh, sneezing, vomiting, and so forth, should be used for making estimates of the need for more drug.

Maintenance Treatment During Rehabilitation

The prophylactic use of methadone for rehabilitating narcotic addicts is one of the more exciting developments in drug therapy of the past decade. The principle involved is the deliberate substitution of one addicting drug by another which has less euphoriant effect and blocks those effects of heroin. Presumably, drug-seeking behavior will be diminished, or at least continued use of heroin will become unrewarding. The pharmacologic basis for this treatment has been reviewed elsewhere (79).

Results from methadone maintenance programs have been variable, but mostly favorable. As heroin addiction has a fairly high mortality and an enormous social morbidity, any approach as promising as methadone maintenance should be fully exploited. Some of the drawbacks to wide-spread application have been the great amount of medical and paramedical resources needed to carry out present treatment programs. More simplified techniques of treatment, including one which would use a longer-acting substitute, dl-acetylmethadol, three times weekly rather than daily doses of methadone, may facilitate the extension of this form of treatment (114). The possibilities for sharply reducing the numbers of heroin addicts are great, but the problem will not be solved by medical means alone.

Besides longer-acting methadone-like drugs, an extensive search is underway for other non-narcotic drugs which might act to block the effects of heroin and lessen drug hunger. The desiderata of such drugs is that they be long-acting, orally active, lack narcotic agonist effects, and be relatively cheap. None presently meets these requirements.

Overdoses of Narcotics

Fatal overdoses of narcotics make opiate dependence a highly dangerous practice. An effective narcotic antagonist, naloxone, rapidly reverses the respiratory depression that leads to a fatal outcome. Early diagnosis is essential, for once full-blown pulmonary edema develops, the situation becomes virtually irretrievable. In using naloxone, one must be aware of the fact that it is a comparatively short-acting drug, while the large dose of narcotic may persist for many hours. Monitoring of patients must be intense, even when their initial responses seem to be quite favorable. If vigilance is relaxed, the patient may quickly slip back into respiratory failure and die before treatment can be resumed. Besides overdoses of narcotics, many other medical complications constitute a threat to the life of a narcotic user (216).

SUMMARY

A diagnosis of one of the psychoses associated with old age should not be made casually as some of these syndromes are manifestations of remediable illnesses. Drug therapy for true psychoses of old age is entirely symptomatic. It may include tricyclic antidepressants for depressive syndromes, phenothiazines for disordered behavior and thinking, and sedative-hypnotic antianxiety drugs as indicated and as tolerated. The principles for treating alcohol withdrawal states are to replace alcohol with a pharmacologically equivalent drug, such as chlordiazepoxide or pentobarbital sodium, and then reduce doses gradually. Aversive therapy of alcoholism with drugs has had only limited success. Management of sedative-hypnotic abuse is entirely similar to that of alcohol abuse, and like the latter, should include social and psychological rehabilitation. Opiate abuse is best managed at present by methadone substitution treatment. Possibly narcotic antagonists might be useful in the future. Social rehabilitation measures are of extreme importance in treating these patients, who usually suffer from severe socioeconomic problems and the residuals of a life of crime or prostitution.

CHAPTER 8

PSYCHOTHERAPEUTIC DRUGS AS MODELS

Historically, advances in psychopharma-cology have been made almost exclusively through empirical, naturalistic, or clinical observations. Despite the recent infusion of more refined scientific methods, it would seem that new treatments might continue to arise in this way. Brash as it may sound, a major goal for the clinical psychopharmacologist should be in developing hypotheses about drug-mind relationships and testing them in clinical trials. From prehistoric times when some genius noted the curious effect on the senses of drinking juices from fermented plants, to the incidental clinical observations of the unique properties of chlorpromazine and reserpine, observers of human behavior have made the major contributions to this field. Clinical hunches — hypotheses, if you will — have advanced other psychiatric treatment as well. The proposal of a large unconscious mental life was such a hunch. So was the possible antagonism between seizures and schizophrenia, which even though probably wrong, was productive of electroconvulsive therapy. Malaria therapy for paresis evolved from the observation that this disease was ameliorated in those patients who managed to survive typhus fever. As in all fields of science, big discoveries come more from relating facts than from finding facts. In psychiatry, the clinician is still best qualified for such a function.

Since I first expressed these thoughts, thirteen years ago, it has not come out quite that way. In the past thirteen years, it has been extremely disappointing that whereas we have many new chemicals, we have had few new drugs. We have developed more models, I suppose, than advances in treatment. So this is the paradox upon which we are caught. We are both blessed and cursed that in psychopharmacology we had a treatment before we had a science. The successful application of drugs to treat schizophrenia, depression, and mania preceded any notion about how they worked. That situation is not unique to clinical psychopharmacology; other clinical pharmacologists live with this paradox, too. But we suffer an additional handicap: we know very little, indeed, about the pathogenesis of the disorders that we are treating.

In this respect, drugs used as treatments have been equally useful as tools for explaining the nature of the disorders. For instance, many years ago, in writing a review of complications from psychotherapeutic drugs, I hazarded the guess that good uses might be made of adversity. The induction of depression in some normal subjects treated briefly with small doses of reserpine seemed to provide a promising model for identifying those patients prone to pathologic depression. This observation of clinical depression from reserpine was the true beginning of the norepinephrine hypothesis of affective disorders, based upon an unpredictable, at least at that time, clinical side effect. I was also struck by the resemblance between drug-induced and naturally-occurring Parkinson's disease, and raised the question: Will the drug-induced disorder advance physiologic understanding of Parkinson's disease and hasten the development of new therapeutic procedures? Now we have levodopa as treatment for Parkinson's disease.

One of my favorite bete noires has been the notion of a model psychosis. Much biochemical research in schizophrenia in the last twenty years has been based on the model psychosis hypothesis. The great mental changes produced by minute amounts of lysergic acid diethylamide (LSD) made a chemical cause for psychosis more feasible than ever before. A great deal of the investigation of LSD and other hallucinogens has assumed that the mental state which they induce has direct relevance to schizophrenia. To some of us, the clinical appearance of the two mental states is so different as to resemble each other no more than do pulmonary tuberculosis and bronchogenic carcinoma. They may share some common characteristics, but the entire ensemble of clinical manifestations is so different that a skilled clinician would have little difficulty in making the differential diagnosis. To others, the perceptual disorder and heightened arousal which these drugs evoke are viewed as highly analogous to the incipient stages, at least, of schizophrenia. Oneiric states in schizophrenia were quite rare a few years back. Recent experience with schizophrenic patients who have used hallucinogens has changed many of the presenting symptoms of schizophrenia. Yet the closer resemblance of schizophrenia today to hallucinogenic drug-induced states may be more a reflection of the highly topical content of schizophrenic delusions than proof for their common pathogenetic mechanism. The resemblances, or lack thereof, between drug-induced model psychosis and schizophrenia are less important than some practical problems regarding the assumptions underlying these chemical theories. What is generally postulated is an endogenous material, continually produced, highly specific in its action in minute doses, for which tolerance does not develop. The latter is quite crucial, as most materials readily produce tolerance.

Few of us would dismiss the possibility of an underlying chemical cause for schizophrenia; on the contrary we strongly believe in it. Although the transmethylation of dopamine hypothesis of two decades ago still has a flicker of life left, it is more due to the role of dopamine than to the process of transmethylation. Once again, the leads implicating dopamine with schizophrenia come from clinical experience with drugs. The two unique pharmacologic properties of antipsychotic drugs – that of evoking in man a syndrome quite like that of Parkinson's disease – and that of ameliorating schizophrenia, now seem to be mediated in large part by a postsynaptic block of dopaminergic receptors. The recent widespread social use of amphetamines has produced a model of paranoid schizophrenia surpassing that of the psychotomimetics. The amphetamine psychosis, too, appears to be mediated through the effects of the drug on dopamine uptake. Finally, the clinical use of levodopa has produced a variety of psychiatric disorders. Our experience a few years ago in treating depressed patients with levodopa convinced me that it was a good way to make them crazy. We quit our investigations after treating five patients. We followed them by treating some schizophrenic patients with levodopa, while maintaining other treatment, and found that a number of patients became worse. Because of the great difficulty in ascertaining whether one was truly affecting symptoms of schizophrenia, it seemed necessary to make the most careful possible study to assure that this was indeed the case. Others have observed schizophrenic-like symptoms from levodopa, as well as those of delirium, depression, and mania. So the picture is far from clear. More recently, two seemingly unrelated but similar neurologic disorders — the choreiform motions from prolonged levodopa treatment of Parkinson's disease and late-appearing dyskinesias following antipsychotic drugs — also seem to share a common dopaminergic mechanism.

The puzzling effects of lithium in affective disorders may make us revise our notions of their etiological bases as we learn more about the mode of action of this drug. Indeed, we should extensively reinvestigate the mode of action of electroconvulsive therapy, which has been effective not only in depression but also in mania. If lithium proves to be a prophylactic treatment against manic-depressive disorder, as now seems highly likely, it will be the first instance of a chemical prophylaxis for a "functional" psychiatric disorder.

Another approach to prophylaxis might be through the identification of persons at risk of developing mental disorders. Because of its possible role in the late-appearing dyskinesias, tests are underway to use challenge doses of levodopa to identify carriers of the gene for Huntington's chorea. Should levodopa be confirmed as a way to exacerbate various psychiatric disorders (mania or schizophrenia) in subjects with a genetic predisposition, the possibility would arise of using similar challenge doses to identify those at risk. We might then be in a position, for the very first time, to practice a preventive psychiatry, which might not only include drug treatment but possibly also alterations in the patient's life style.

The revolution in psychiatry that effective psychotherapeutic drugs started less than two decades ago will continue for a great many years more. Our hope as psychopharmacologists is that it will unravel some of the mysteries of mental disorders and lead to their still more effective treatment.

REFERENCES

1. Abdulla, Y. H., and Hamadah, K.: 3', 5' cyclic adenosine monophosphate in depression and mania. Lancet, 1:378, 1970.
2. Adelson, D., and Epstein, L. J.: A study of phenothiazines with male and female chronically ill schizophrenic patients. J. Nerv Ment Dis, 134:543, 1962.
3. Alderton, H. R.: A review of childhood schizophrenia. Can Psychiatr Assoc J, 11:276, 1966.
4. Alexander, C. S., and Nino, A.: Cardiovascular complications in young patients taking psychotropic drugs. Am Heart J, 78:757, 1969.
5. Alexandris, A., and Lundell, F. W.: Effect of thioridazine, amphetamine and placebo on the hyperkinetic syndrome and cognitive area in mentally deficient children. Can Med Assoc J, 98:92, 1968.
6. Angst, J., Weis, P., Grof, P., Baastrup, P. C., and Schou, M.: Lithium prophylaxis in recurrent affective disorders. Br J Psychiatr, 116:604, 1970.
7. Asberg, M., Cronholm, B., Sjoquist, F., and Tuck, D.: Relationship between plasma level and therapeutic effect on nortriptyline. Br Med J, 3:331, 1971.
8. Axelrod, J.: Amphetamine: metabolism, physiological disposition and its effects on catecholamine storage. In Casta, E., and Garattini, S. (Eds.): Amphetamine and Related Compounds. New York, Raven Press, 1970, p. 207.
9. Axelrod, J.: Noradrenaline: Fate and control of its biosynthesis. Science, 173:598, 1971.
10. Baastrup, P. C., and Schou, M.: Lithium as a prophylactic agent. Its effect against recurrent depressions and manic-depressive psychosis. Arch Gen Psychiatr, 16:162, 1967.
11. Baastrup, P. C., Poulsen, J. V., Schou, M. Thomsen, K., and Amdisen, A.: Prophylactic lithium. Double-blind discontinuation in manic-depressive and recurrent depressive disorders. Lancet, 2:326, 1970.
12. Baer, R. L., and Harber, L. C.: Photosensitivity induced by drugs. JAMA, 192:989-990, 1965.
13. Ball, J. A. C., and Taylor, A. R.: Effect of cyclandelate on mental function and cerebral blood flow in elderly patients. Lancet, 3:525, 1967.
14. Ban, T. A., and Lehmann, H. E.: Nicotinic acid in the treatment of schizophrenias. Canadian Mental Health Association Collaborative

Study. Progress report I. Can Ment Health Assoc, Toronto, 1970, pp. 1-18.

15. Barcel, N. A.: Clinical experience with a new type of antidepressant drug: Ditran. J. Neuropsychiat, 2:271, 1961.
16. Berger, F.: The relation between the pharmacological properties of meprobamate and the clinical usefulness of the drug. In Efron, D. H. (Ed.): Psychopharmacology. A Review of Progress. 1957-1967. Public Health Service Publication No. 1836, U. S. Govt. Printing Office, Washington, D. C., 1960. pp. 139-152.
17. Berger, F. M.: Mental disease and drugs affecting it. Perspect Biol Med, 13:31, 1969.
18. Bickel, M. H., and Weder, H. J.: The total fate of a drug: Kinetics of distribution, excretion, and formation of 14 metabolites in rats treated with imipramine. Arch Int Pharmacodyn Ther, 173:433, 1968.
19. Blackwell, B., Marley, E., Price, J., and Taylor, E.: Hypertensive interactions between monoamine oxidase inhibitors and foodstuff. Br J Psychiatr, 113:349, 1967.
20. Blackwell, B., and Shepherd, M.: Prophylactic lithium: Another therapeutic myth? An examination of evidence to date. Lancet, 1:968, 1968.
21. Bradley, C.: The behavior of children receiving benzedrine. Am J Psychiatr, 94:577, 1937.
22. Brill, N. Q., Koegler, R. R., Epstein, L. J., and Forgy, E. W.: Controlled study of psychiatric outpatient treatment. Arch Gen Psychiatr, 10:581-595, 1964.
23. Brodie, B. B., Dick, P., Kielholz, P., Poeldinger, W., and Theobald, W.: Preliminary pharmacological and clinical results with desmethyl-imipramine (DMI, G-35020), a metabolite of imipramine. Psychopharmacologia, 2:467, 1961.
24. Brodie, H. K. H., Murphy, D. L., Goodwin, F. K., and Bunney, W. E., Jr.: Catecholamines and mania: The effect of alphamethylparatyrosine on manic behavior and catecholamine metabolism. Clin Pharmacol Ther, 12:218, 1971.
25. Bunney, W. E., Janowsky, D. S., Goodwin, F. K., Davis, J. M., Brodie, H. K. H., Murphy, D. L., and Chase, T. N.: Effect of l-dopa on depression. Lancet 1:885, 1969.
26. Burn, J. H.: Tyramine and other amines as noradrenaline-releasing substances. In Wolstenholme, G. E. W. O'Connor, M. and Vane, J. R. (Eds): Adrenergic Mechanisms. London, J. A. Churchill, Ltd., 1960. p. 326.
27. Caffey, E. M., Jr., Diamond, L. S., Frank, T. V., Grasberger, J. C., Herman, L., Klett, C. J., and Rothstein, C.: Discontinuation or reduction of chemotherapy in chronic schizophrenics. J Chron Dis, 17:347, 1964.
28. Caldwell, H. C., Westlake, W. J., Connor, S. M. and Flanagen, T.: A

pharmacokinetic analysis of lithium carbonate absorption from several formulations in man. J Clin Pharmacol, 11:349, 1971.

29. Carter, C. H.: Nortriptyline HCl as a tranquilizer for disturbed mentally retarded patients: A controlled study. Am J. Sci, 251:465, 1966.

30. Casey, J. F., Bennett, I. F., Lindley, C. J., Hollister, L. E., Gordon, M. H., and Springer, N. N.: Drug therapy in schizophrenia: A controlled study of the relative effectiveness of chlorpromazine, promazine, phenobarbital, and placebo. Arch Gen Psychiatr, 2:210, 1960.

31. Casey, J. F., Lasky, J. J., Klett, C. J., and Hollister, L. E.: Treatment of schizophrenic reactions with phenothiazine derivatives: A comparative study of chlorpromazine, triflupromazine, mepazine, prochlorperazine, perphenazine, and phenobarbital. Am. J Psychiatr, 117, 1960.

32. Casey, J. F., Hollister, L. E., Klett, C. J., Lasky, J. J. and Caffey, E. M., Jr.: Combined drug therapy of chronic schizophrenics: A controlled evaluation of placebo, dextroamphetamine, imipramine, isocarboxazid, and trifluoperazine added to maintenance doses of chlorpromazine. Am J Psychiatr, 117:997, 1961.

33. Cattell, R. B., and Scheier, I. H.: Handbook for the IPAT Anxiety Scale Questionnaire. Champaign, Ill., Institute for Personality and Ability Testing, 1966.

34. Christensen, E., Moller, J. E., and Faurbye, A.: Neuropathological investigation of 28 brains from patients with dyskinesia. Acta Psychiatr Scand, 46:14, 1970.

35. Clemens, T. L., and Selesnick, S. T.: Psychological method for evaluating medication by repeated exposure to a stressor film. Dis Nerv Syst, 28:98-104, 1967.

36. Clinical Psychiatry Committee of the Medical Res. Council. Clinical trial of the treatment of depressive illness. Br Med J 1:881, 1965.

37. Colburn, R. W., Goodwin, F. K., Bunney, W. E., Jr., and Davis, J. M.: Effect of lithium on the uptake of noradrenaline by synaptosomes. Nature, 215:1395, 1967.

38. Conners, C. K., and Eisenberg, L.: The effects of methylphenidate on symptomatology and learning in disturbed children. Am J Psychiatr, 120:48, 1963.

39. Conners, C. K., Rothschild, G., Eisenberg, L., Schwartz, L. S., and Robinson, E.: Dextroamphetamine sulfate in children with learning disorders. Arch Gen Psychiatr, 21:182, 1969.

40. Conney, A. H.: Pharmacological implications of microsomal enzyme induction. Pharmacol Rev, 19:317-366, 1967.

41. Coppen, A., Shaw, D. M., Malleson, A., and Costain, R.: Mineral metabolism in mania. Br Med J, 1:71-75, 1966.

42. Coppen, A., Noguera, R., Bailey, J., Burns, B. H., Swani, M., Hare, E. H., Gardner, R., and Maags, R.: Prophylactic lithium in affective disorders. Controlled trial. Lancet, 2:275, 1971.

43. Coppen, A.: Biogenic amines and affective disorders. In Ho, B. T., and

174   *Clinical Use of Psychotherapeutic Drugs*

McIsaac, W. M. (Eds): Brain Chemistry and Mental Disease. New York, Plenum Press, 1971. p. 123.

44. Council on Mental Health. Narcotics and medical practice. Medical use of morphine and morphine-like drugs and management of persons dependent on them. JAMA, 218:578, 1971.

45. Court, J. H., and Mai, F. M. M. M.: A double-blind intensive crossover design trial of methysergide in mania. Med J Australia, 2:526, 1970.

46. Crane, G. E., and Naranjo, E. R.: Motor disorders induced by neuroleptics. Arch Gen Psychiatr, 24:179, 1971.

47. Cunningham, M. A., Pillai, V., and Blackford-Rogers, W. J.: Haloperidol in the treatment of children with severe behavior disorders. Br J Psychiat, 114:845, 1968.

48. Curry, S. H., Marshall, J. H. L., Davis, J. M., and Janowsky, D. S.: Chlorpromazine plasma levels and effects. Arch Gen Psychiatr, 22:289, 1970.

49. Curry, S. H.: Chlorpromazine: Concentrations in plasma, excretion in urine and duration of effect. Proc Royal Soc Med, 64:285, 1971.

50. Davies, B., Carroll, B. J., and Mowbray, R. M.: Depressive Illness. Some Research Studies. Springfield, Ill., Charles C Thomas, 1972, pp. 23-208.

51. Davis, J. M., Bartlett, E., and Termini, B. A.: Overdosage of psychotropic drugs: A review. Dis Nerv Syst, 29:157-246, 1968.

52. Davis, J. M., and Fann, W. E.: Lithium. Ann Rev. Pharmacol, 11:285, 1971.

53. Davis, V. E., and Walsh, M. J.: Alcohol, amines and alkaloids: A possible biochemical basis for alcohol addiction. Science, 167:1005, 1970.

54. Dingell, J. V., Salser, F., and Gillette, J. R.: Species differences in the metabolism of imipramine and desmethylimipramine (DMI). J Pharmacol Exp Ther, 143:14, 1964.

55. Edwards, G.: Comparison of the effects of imipramine and desipramine on some symptoms of depressive illness. Br J Psychiatr, 111:889, 1965.

56. Efron, S. H., Harris, S. R., Manian, A. A., and Gaudette, L. D.: Levels of extractable and bound chlorpromazine and some of its metabolites in animals and human plasma (in press).

57. Eisenberg, L.: Role of drugs in treating disturbed children. Children, 11:167, 1964.

58. Engelhardt, D. M., Rosen, B., Freedman, N., and Margolis, R.: Phenothiazines in prevention of psychiatric hospitalization. IV. Delay or prevention of hospitalization – a re-evaluation. Arch Gen Psychiatr, 16:98-101, 1967.

59. Epstein, L. C., Lasagna, L., Connors, C. K., and Rodriquez, A.: Correlation of dextroamphetamine excretion and drug response in hyperkinetic children. J Nerv Ment Dis, 146:136, 1968.

60. Eveloff, H. H.: Psychopharmacologic agents in child psychiatry. Arch Gen Psychiatr, 14:472-481, 1966.

61. Eveloff, H. H.: Pediatric psychopharmacology. In Clark, W. G., and del Giudice, J.(Eds): Principles of Psychopharmacology. New York, Academic Press, 1970. pp. 683-694.
62. Feighner, J. P., King, L. J., Schuckit, M. A., Croughan, J., and Briscoe, W.: Hormonal potentiation of imipramine and ECT in primary depression. Am J Psychiatr, 128:1230, 1972.
63. Fieve, R. R., Platman, S., and Plutchik, R.: The use of lithium in affective disorders. I. Acute endogenous depression. Am J Psychiatr, 125:487, 1968.
64. Fink, M., Klein, D. F., and Kramer, J. C.: Clinical efficacy of chlorpromazine-procyclidine combination, imipramine and placebo in depressive disorders. Psychopharmacologia, 7:27, 1965.
65. Fink, M., Simeon, J., Itil, T. M., and Freedman, A. M.: Clinical antidepressant activity of cyclazocine. Clin Pharmacol Ther, 11:41, 1970.
66. Fish, B.: Problems of diagnosis and the definition of comparable groups: A neglected issue in drug research with children. Am J Psychiatr, 125:72, 1969.
67. Forrest, I. S., Bolt, A. G., and Serra, M. T.: Distribution of chlorpromazine metabolites in selected organs of psychiatric patients chronically dosed up to the time of death. Biochem Pharmacol, 17:2061, 1968.
68. Forrest, I. S., Forrest, F. M., and Serra, M. T.: Chlorpromazine retention. Am J Psychiatr, 126:271, 1969.
69. Frommer, E. A.: Treatment of childhood depression with anti-depressant drugs. Br Med J, 1:729, 1967.
70. Fry, D. E., and Marks, V.: Value of plasma-lithium monitoring. Lancet, 1:886, 1971.
71. Galbrecht, C. R., and Klett, C. J.: Predicting response to phenothiazines: The right drug for the right patient. J Nerv Ment Dis, 147:173-183, 1968.
72. Gallant, D. D., Bishop, M. P., Guerrero-Figuero, R., Selby, M., and Phillips, R.: Doxepin versus diazepam. A controlled evaluation in 100 chronic alcoholic patients. J Clin Pharmacol, 9:57, 1969.
73. Gen. Practitioner Research Group. Oxazepam in anxiety. Practitioner (London), 199:1191, 1967.
74. Gen. Practitioner Research Group. Chlordiazepoxide with amitriptyline in neurotic depression (Report No. 134). Practitioner (London), 202:437-440, 1969.
75. Gershon, E. S., Dunner, D. L., and Goodwin, F. K.: Towards a biology of the affective disorders. Arch Gen Psychiatr, 25:1, 1971.
76. Gershon, S.: Lithium in mania. Clin Pharmacol Ther, 11:168, 1970.
77. Goldberg, S. C., Frisch, W. A., Drossman, A. K., Schooler, N. R., and Johnson, G. F. S.: Prediction of response to phenothiazines in schizophrenia. A cross-validation study. Arch Gen Psychiatr, 26:367, 1972.

78. Goldfield, M., and Weinstein, M. R.: Lithium in pregnancy: A review with recommendations. Am J Psychiatr, 127:888, 1971.
79. Goldstein, A.: Heroin addiction and the role of methadone in its treatment. Arch Gen Psychiatr, 26:291, 1972.
80. Goldstein, B. J., and Brauzer, B.: Pharmacological considerations in the treatment of anxiety and depression in medical practice. Med Clin North Am, 55:485-494, 1971.
81. Goodwin, F. K., Brodie, H. K. H., Murphy, D. L., and Bunney, W. E., Jr.: L-dopa, catecholamines and behavior: A clinical and biochemical study in depressed patients. Biol Psychiatr, 2:341, 1970.
82. Gorham, D. R., and Pokorny, A. D.: Effects of a phenothiazine and/or group psychotherapy with schizophrenics. Dis Nerv Syst, 25:77, 1964.
83. Gram, L. F., and Overo, K. F.: Drug interaction: Inhibitory effect of neuroleptics on metabolism of tricyclic antidepressants in man. Br Med J, 1:463, 1972.
84. Granville-Grossman, K. L., and Turner, P.: The effect of propranolol on anxiety. Lancet, 1:788, 1966.
85. Greenblatt, M., Grosser, G. H., and Wechsler, H.: Differential response of hospitalized depressed patients to somatic therapy. Am J Psychiatr, 120:935, 1964.
86. Grinspoon, L., Ewalt, J. R., and Shader, R.: Long-term treatment of chronic schizophrenia. Int J Psychiatr, 4:116, 1967.
87. Grof, P., and Vinar, O.: Combination of nortriptyline and amitriptyline in depression. An intensive and controlled study. Activitas Nervosa Superior (Praha), 8:380-381, 1966.
88. Gundlach, R., Engelhardt, D. M., Hankoff, L., Paley, H., Rudorfer, L., and Bird, E.: A double-blind outpatient study of diazepam (Valium®) and placebo. Psychopharmacologia, 9:81, 1966.
89. Gyermek, L.: The pharmacology of imipramine and related anti-depressants. Int Rev Neurobiol, 9:95, 1966.
90. Hammar, C. G., Holmstedt, B., Lindgren, J. E., and Tham, R.: The combination of gas chromatography and mass spectrometry in the identification of drugs and metabolites. Adv Pharmacol Chemother, 7:53, 1969.
91. Hanlon, T. E., Ota, K. Y., Agallianos, D. D., Berman, S. A., Bethon, G. D., Kobler, F., and Kurland, A. A.: Combined drug treatment of newly hospitalized, acutely ill psychiatric patients. Dis Nerv Syst, 30:104, 1969.
92. Hanlon, T. E., Ota, K. Y., and Kurland, A. A.: Comparative effects of fluphenazine, fluphenazine-chlordiazepoxide and fluphenazine-imipramine. Dis Nerv Syst, 31:171-176, 1970.
93. Haskovec, L., and Rysanek, K.: Die wirkung von lithium auf den metabolismus der katecholamine und indolalkylamine beim menschen. Arzenimittelforschung, 19:426, 1969.
94. Heston, L. L.: The genetics of schizophrenic and schizoid disease.

Science, 167:249, 1970.
95. Holden, J. M. C., Itil, T. M., Keskiner, A., and Fink, M.: Thioridazine and chlordiazepoxide, alone and combined, in the treatment of chronic schizophrenia. Comprehens. Psychiatr, 9:633-643, 1968.
96. Hollister, L. E., Jones, K. P., Brownfield, B., and Johnson, F.: Chlorpromazine alone and with reserpine. Calif Med, 83:218-221, 1955.
97. Hollister, L. E., and Glazener, F. S.: Withdrawal reaction from mebrobamate alone and combined with promazine: A controlled study. Psychopharmacologia, 1:336-341, 1970.
98. Hollister, L. E., Motzenbecker, F. P., and Degan, R. O.: Withdrawal reactions from chlordiazepoxide (Librium®). Psychopharmacologia, 2:63-68, 1961.
99. Hollister, L. E., Overall, J. E., Meyer, F., and Shelton, J.: Perphenazine combined with amitriptyline in newly-admitted schizophrenics. Am J Psychiatr, 120:571-578, 1963.
100. Hollister, L. E., Overall, J. E., Johnson, M., Pennington, V., Katz, G., and Shelton, J.: Controlled comparison of amitriptyline, imipramine and placebo in hospitalized depressed patients. J Nerv Ment Dis, 139:370, 1964.
101. Hollister, L. E.: Complications from psychotherapeutic drugs. Clin Pharmacol Ther, 5:322, 1964.
102. Hollister, L. E., and Levy, G.: Kinetics of meprobamate elimination in humans. Chemotherapia, 9:20-24, 1964.
103. Hollister, L. E., Overall, J. E., Shelton, J. Pennington, V., Kimbell, I., and Johnson, M.: Drug therapy of depression. Amitriptyline, perphenazine and their combination in different syndromes. Arch Gen Psychiatr, 17:486, 1967.
104. Hollister, L. E., Overall, J. E., Bennett, J. L., Kimbell, I., and Shelton, J.: Specific therapeutic actions of acetophenazine, perphenazine and benzquinamide in newly-admitted schizophrenic patients. Clin Pharmacol Ther, 8:249-255, 1957.
105. Hollister, L. E.: Clinical use of psychotherapeutic drugs. Current status. Clin Pharmacol Ther, 10:170, 1969.
106. Hollister, L. E.: Toxicology of psychotherapeutic drugs. In Clark, W. G., and del Guidice, J. (Eds.): Principles of Psychopharmacology. New York, Academic Press, 1970, pp. 537-546.
107. Hollister, L. E., Curry, S. H., Derr, J. E., and Kanter, S. L.: Studies of delayed-action medication. V. Plasma levels and urinary excretion of chlorpromazine in four different dosage forms given acutely and in steadystate conditions. Clin Pharmacol Ther, 11:49, 1970.
108. Hollister, L. E., and Curry, S. H.: Urinary excretion of chlorpromazine metabolites following single doses and in steady-state conditions. Research Comm Chem Pathol Pharmacol, 2:330, 1971.
109. Hollister, L. E., Overall, J. E., Pokorny, A. D., and Shelton, J.: Acetophenazine and diazepam in anxious depressions. Arch Gen

Psychiatr, 24:273, 1971.
110. Hordern, A.: Psychiatry and the tranquilizers. New Eng J Med, 265:584-634, 1961.
111. Hullin, R. P., Swinscoe, J. C., McDonald, R., and Dransfield, G. A.: Metabolic balance studies on the effect of lithium salts in manic-depressive psychosis. Br J Psychiatr, 114:1561, 1968.
112. Idanpaan-Heikkila, J. E., Taska, R. J., Allen, H. A., and Schollar, J. C.: Placental transfer of diazepam-^{14}C in mice, hamsters and monkeys. J Pharmacol Exp Ther, 176:752, 1971.
113. Irwin, S.: Antineurotics: Practical pharmacology of the sedative-hypnotics and minor tranquilizers. In Efron, D. F. (Ed.): Psychopharmacology. A Review of Progress. 1957-1967. Public Health Service Publication No. 1836, U. S. Govt. Printing Office Washington, 1968. pp. 185-204.
114. Jaffe, J. H., and Senay, E. C.: Methadone and 1-methadyl acetate. Use in management of narcotics addicts JAMA, 216:1303, 1971.
115. Janecek, J., Vestre, N. D., Schiele, B. C., and Zimmerman, R.: Oxazepam in the treatment of anxiety states: A controlled study. J Psychiatr, Res, 4:199, 1966.
116. Janssen, P. A. J.: Chemical and pharmacological classification of neuroleptics. In Bokon, O. P., Janssen, P. A. J., and Bokon, J. (Eds): Modern Problems in Pharmacopsychiatry: The Neuroleptics. Vol. 5 Basel, S. Karger, 1970, pp. 34-44.
117. Jenner, F. A., and Kerry, R. J.: Comparison of diazepam, chlordiazepoxide and amylobarbitane (a multidose double-blind cross-over study). Dis Nerv Syst, 28:245-249, 1967.
118. Johnson, G., Gershon, S., Burdock, E. I., Floyd, A., and Hekemian, L.: Comparative effects of lithium and chlorpromazine in the treatment of acute manic states. Br J Psychiatr, 119:267, 1971.
119. Jori, A., Prestini, P. E., and Pugliatti, C.: Effect of diazepam and chlordiazepoxide on the metabolism of other drugs. J Pharm Pharmacol, 21:387, 1969.
120. Kaim, S. C., Klett, C. J., and Rothfeld, B.: Treatment of the acute alcohol withdrawal state: A comparison of four drugs. Am J Psychiatr, 125:1640-1646, 1969.
121. Kaim, S. C., and Klett, C. J.: Treatment of delirium tremens. A comparative evaluation of four drugs. Q J Studies Alcohol, in press.
122. Kales, A., Malmstrom, E. J., Scharf, M. B., and Rubin, R. T.: Psycholphysiological and biochemical changes following use and withdrawal of hypnotics. In Kales, A. (Ed.): Sleep, Physiology and Pathology. Philadelphia, J. B. Lippincott, 1969, pp. 331-343.
123. Kaplan, R., Blume, S., Rosenberg, S., Pitrelli, J., and Turner, W. J.: Phenytoin, metronidazole and multivitamins in the treatment of alcoholism. Q J Studies of Alcohol, 33:97, 1972.
124. Kelly, D., Brown, C. C., and Shafter, J. W.: A controlled physiological,

clinical and psychological evaluation of chlordiazepoxide. Br J Psychiatr, 115:1387-1392, 1969.

125. Kiloh, L. G., and Garside, R. F.: The independence of neurotic depression and endogenous depression. Br J Psychiatr, 109:451, 1963.

126. Klett, C. J., and Caffey, E. M., Jr.: Weight changes during treatment with phenothiazine derivatives. J Neuropsychiatr, 2:102-108, 1960.

127. Klett, C. J., Hollister, L. E., Caffey, E. M. Jr., and Kaim, S. C.: Evaluating changes in symptoms during acute alcohol withdrawal. Arch Gen Psychiatr, 24:174, 1971.

128. Klett, C. J., and Caffey, E. M., Jr. Evaluation of the long-term need for antiparkinson drugs by chronic schizophrenics. Arch Gen Psychiatr, 26:374, 1972.

129. Kline, N. S.: Depression: Diagnosis and treatment. Med Clin North Am, 45:1041, 1961.

130. Knobel, M., Wolman, M. B., and Mason, E.: Hyperkineasia and organicity in children. Arch Gen Psychiatr, 1:310, 1959.

131. Kuhn, R.: The treatment of depressive states with G 22355 (imipramine hydrochloride). Am J Psychiatr, 115:459, 1958.

132. Kusumi, Y.: A cutaneous side effect of lithium: Report of two cases. Dis Nerv Syst, 32:853-854, 1971.

133. Lader, M. H., and Wing, L.: Physiological measures sedative drugs, and morbid anxiety. In Maudsley Monograph No. 14. London, Oxford University Press, 1966, pp. 1-167.

134. Lasagna, L., and Epstein, K. C.: The use of amphetamines in the treatment of hyperkinetic children. In Costa, E., and Garattini, S. (Eds.): International Symposium on Amphetamines and Related Compounds. New York, Raven Press, 1970, pp. 849-864.

135. Lasky, J. J., Klett, C. J., Caffey, E. M., Jr., Bennett, J. L., Rosenblum, M. P., and Hollister, L. E.: Drug treatemnt of schizophrenic patients: A comparative evaluation of chlorpromazine, chlorprothixene, fluphenazine, reserpine, thioridazine, and triflupromazine. Dis Nerv Syst, 23:698, 1962.

136. Leemsta, J. E., and Koenig, K. L.: Sudden death and phenothiazines. A current controversy. Arch Gen Psychiatr, 18:137, 1968.

137. Leff, J. P., and Wing, J. K.: Trial of maintenance therapy in schizophrenia. Br Med J, 3:599, 1971.

138. Lehmann, H. E., Cahn, C. H., and DeVerteuil, R. L.: The treatment of depressive conditions with imipramine (G 22355). Can Psychiatr Assoc J, 3:155, 1958.

139. Lehmann, H. E., Ananth, J. V., Geagea, K. C.: Treatment of depression with dexedrine and demerol. Curr Ther Res, 13:42, 1971.

140. Lennard, H. L., Epstein, L. J., Bernstein, A., and Ransom, D. C.: Hazards implicit in prescribing psychoactive drugs. Science, 169:438, 1970.

141. Lorr, M., McNair, D. M., Weinstein, G. J., Michaux, W. M., and Raskin,

A.: Meprobamate and chlorpromazine in psychotherapy. Arch Gen Psychiatr, 4:381-389, 1961.
142. Lorr, M., McNair, D. M., and Weinstein, G. J.; Early effects of chlordiazepoxide (Librium) used with psychotherapy. J Psychiatr Res, 1:257-270, 1963.
143. Lorr, M., and Klett, J.: Psychotic behavioral types. A cross-cultural comparison. Arch Gen Psychiatr, 20:592, 1969.
144. Lowenstein, L., Simone, R., Boulter, P., and Nathan, P.: Effect of fructose on alcohol concentrations in the blood of man. JAMA, 213:1889, 1970.
145. Lundwall, L., and Baekeland, F.: Disulfiram treatment of alcoholism. J Nerv Ment Dis, 153:381, 1971.
146. Lynn, E. J., Satloff, A., and Tinling, D. C.: Mania and the use of lithium: A three-year study. Am J Psychiatr, 127:96, 1971.
147. Maas, J. W., Fawcett, J. A., and Dekirmenjian, H.: Catecholamine metabolism, depressive illness and drug response. Arch Gen Psychiatr, 26:252, 1972.
148. Malitz, S., and Kanzler, M.: Are antidepressants better than placebo? Am J Psychiatr, 127:1605, 1971.
149. Mannheimer, D. I., Mellinger, G. D., and Balter, M. B.: Psychotherapeutic drugs. Use among adults in California. Calif Med, 109:445, 1968.
150. Martin, W. R., Sloan, J. W., Sapira, J. D., and Jasinski, D. R.: Physiologic, subjective, and behavioral effects of amphetamine, methamphetamine, ephedrine, phenmetrazine and methylphenidate in man. Clin Pharmacol Ther, 12:245, 1971.
151. May, P. R. A.: Treatment of Schizophrenia. A Comparative Study of Five Treatment Methods. New York, Science House, 1968, pp. 1-352.
152. McDonall, A., Owen S., and Robin, A. A.: A controlled comparison of diazepam and amylobarbitane in anxiety states. Br J Psychiatr, 112:629-631, 1966.
153. McNair, D. M., Goldstein, A. P., Lorr, M., Cibelli, L. A., and Roth, I.: Some effects of chlordiazepoxide and meprobamate with psychiatric outpatients. Psychopharmacologia, 7:256-265, 1965.
154. McReynolds, P. (Ed.): Advances in Psychological Assessment. Chapter XIII. The assessment of anxiety. A survey of available techniques. Palo Alto, Cal., Science and Behavior Books, 1968.
155. Mendels, J.: Relationship between depression and mania. Lancet, 1:342, 1971.
156. Merlis, S., Sheppard, C., Collins, L., and Fiorentino, D.: Polypharmacy in psychiatry: Patterns of differential treatment. Am J Psychiatr, 126:1647-1651, 1970.
157. Michaux, M. H., Hanlon, T. E., Ota, K. Y., and Kurland, A. A.: Phenothiazines in the treatment of newly admitted state hospital patients: Global comparison of eight compounds in terms of an

outcome index. Curr Ther Res, 6:331, 1964.

158. Moody, J. P., Tait, A. C., and Todrick, A.: Plasma levels of imipramine and desmethylimipramine during therapy. Br J Psychiatr, 113:183, 1967.

159. Morrelli, H. F.: Rational therapy of drug over-dosage. In Clinical Pharmacology. Basic Principles in Therapeutics. New York, MacMillan, 1972, pp. 605-623.

160. Mosher, L. R.: Nictonic acid side effects and toxicity: A review. Am J Psychiatr, 126:124, 1970.

161. Muller, C.: The overmedicated society: Forces in the marketplace for medical care. Science, 176:488, 1972

162. National Institute of Mental Health-Psychopharmacology Service Center Collaborative Study Group: Phenothiazine treatment in acute schizophrenia. Arch Gen Psychiatr, 10:246, 1964.

163. Orlov, P., Kasparian, G., Di Mascio, A., and Cole, J. O.: Withdrawal of antiparkinson drugs. Arch Gen Psychiatr, 25:410, 1971.

164. Overall, J. E., and Gorman, D. R.: The brief psychiatric rating scale. Psychol Rep, 10:799, 1962.

165. Overall, J. E., Hollister, L. E., Pokorny, A. D., Casey, J. F., and Katz, G.: Drug therapy in depressions. Clin Pharmacol Ther, 3:16, 1962.

166. Overall, J. E., Hollister, L. E., Meyer, F., Kimbell, I., Jr., and Shelton, J.: Imipramine and thioridazine in depressed and schizophrenic patients. Are there specific antidepressant drugs? JAMA, 189:605, 1964.

167. Overall, J. E., Hollister, L. E., Shelton, J., Johnson, M. H., and Kimbell, I., Jr.: Tranylcypromine compared with dextroamphetamine in hospitalized depressed patients. Dis Nerv Syst, 27:653, 1966.

168. Overall, J. E., Hollister, L. E., Johnson, M., and Pennington, V.: Nosology of depression and differential response to drugs. JAMA 195:946, 1966.

169. Overall, J. E., Hollister, L. E., and Pichot, P.: Major psychiatric disorders. A four-dimensional model. Arch Gen Psychiatr, 16:146, 1967.

170. Paykel, E. S.: Classification of depressed patients: A cluster analysis derived grouping. Br J Psychiatr, 118:275, 1971.

171. Paykel, E. S.: Depressive typologies and response to amitriptyline. Br J Psychiatr, 120:147, 1972.

172. Pillard, R. C., and Fisher, S.: Effects of chlordiazepoxide and secobarbital on film-induced anxiety. Psychopharmacologia, 12:18-23, 1967.

173. Pisciotta, A. V.: Mechanisms of phenothiazine induced agranulocytosis. In Efron, D. (Ed.): Psychopharmacology. A Review of Progress, 1957-1967. Public Health Service Publication No. 1836, U. S. Govt. Printing Office, Washington, 1968. pp. 597-605.

174. Platman, S., Rohrlich, J., and Fieve, R.: Absorption and excretion of

lithium in manic-depressive disease. Dis Nerv Syst, 29:733, 1968.
175. Platman, S. R., and Fieve, R. R.: Biochemical aspects of lithium in affective disorders. Arch Gen Psychiatr, 19:659, 1968.
176. Platman, S. R.: Lithium and rubidium: A role in the affective disorders. Dis Nerv Syst, 32:604, 1971.
177. Platman, S. R., Hilton, J. G., Koss, M. C., and Kelly, W. G.: Production of cortisol in patients with manic-depressive psychosis treated with lithium carbonate. Dis Nerv Syst, 32:542, 1971.
178. Pletscher, A., Shore, P. A., and Brodie, B. B.: Serotonin as mediator of reserpine action in brain. J Pharmacol Exp Ther, 116:84, 1956.
179. Polatin, P., and Fieve, R. R.: Patient rejection of lithium carbonate prophylaxis. JAMA, 218:864, 1971.
180. Pollitt, J., and Young, J.: Anxiety state or masked depression? A study based on the action of monoamine oxidase inhibitors. Br J Psychiatr, 119:143, 1971.
181. Prien, R. F., and Cole, J. O.: High dose chlorpromazine therapy in chronic schizophrenia. Report of NIMH-Psychopharmacology Research Branch Collaborative Study Group. Arch Gen Psychiatr, 18:482-495, 1968.
182. Prien, R. F., Cole, J. O., and Belkin, N. F.: Relapse in chronic schizophrenics following abrupt withdrawal of tranquillizing medication. Br J Psychiatr, 115:679, 1969.
183. Prien, R. F., De Long, S. L., Cole, J. O., and Levine, J.: Ocular changes occurring with prolonged high dose chlorpromazine therapy. Arch Gen Psychiatr, 23:464, 1970.
184. Prien, R. F., Caffey, E. M. Jr., and Klett, C. J.: A comparison of lithium carbonate and chlorpromazine in the treatment of mania. Arch Gen Psychiatr, 26:146, 1972.
185. Prien, R. F., Caffey, E. M. Jr., and Klett, C. J.: The relationship between serum lithium level and clinical response in acute manics treated with lithium carbonate. Br J Psychiatr, 120:409, 1972.
186. Prien, R. F., Caffey, E. M. Jr., and Klett, C. J.: A comparison of lithium carbonate and chlorpromazine in the treatment of excited schizo-affectives (in press).
187. Pritchard, M.: Prognosis of schizophrenia before and after pharmaco-therapy. I. Short term outcome. Br J Psychiatr, 113:1345, 1967; II. Three-year follow up. Ibid., p. 1353.
188. Ramsey, T. A., Mendels, J., Stokes, J. W., and Fitzgerald, R. G.: Lithium carbonate and kidney function. A failure in renal concentrating ability. JAMA, 219:1446, 1972.
189. Randall, L. O., and Schallek, W.: Pharmacological activity of certain benzodiazepines. In Efron, D. H. (Ed.): Psychopharmacology. A Review of Progress. 1957-1967. Public Health Service Publication No. 1836, U. S. Govt. Printing Office, Washington, 1968, pp. 153-184.
190. Raskin, A., Schotterbrandt, J. C., Reatig, N., and McKeon, J. J.:

Differential responses to chlorpromazine, imipramine and placebo. A study of subgroups of hospitalized depressed patients. Arch Gen Psychiatr, 23:164, 1970.

191. Rickels, K., Clark, T. W., Ewing, J. H., Klingensmith, W. C., Morris, H. M. and Smock, C. D. Evaluation of tranquilizing drugs in medical outpatients. Meprobamate, prochlorperazine and amobarbital sodium and placebo. JAMA, 171:1649-1656, 1959.

192. Rickels, K., Raab, I., DeSilverio, R., and Etemad, B.: Drug treatment in depression. Antidepressant or tranquilizer. JAMA, 201:675, 1967.

193. Rickels, K. (Ed.): Non-specific factors in drug therapy of neurotic patients. In Non-Specific Factors in Drug Therapy. Springfield, Ill., Charles C Thomas, 1968, pp. 3-26.

194. Rickels, K.: Drug use in outpatient treatment. Am J Psychiatr, 124:20, 1968.

195. Rifkin, A., Quitkin, R., Carrillo, C., and Klein, D. F.: Very high dosage fluphenazine for nonchronic treatment-refractory patients. Arch Gen Psychiatr, 25:398, 1971.

196. Rizzo, M., Pantarotto, C., Riva, E., Gianelli, A., Morselli, P. L., and Garattini, S.: Interactions of tricyclic antidepressants with other drugs. Paper read at Fifth International Congress of Pharmacology, San Francisco, 1972.

197. Roth, G.: Psychopharmakon hoc est: medicina aminae (1548). Confinia Psychiatrica, 7:179-182, 1964.

198. Rubin, E., and Lieber, C. S.: Alcoholism, alcohol and drugs. Science, 172:1097, 1971.

199. Rutter, M., Lebovici, S., Eisenberg, L., Sneznevskij, A. V., Sadoun, R., Brooke, E., and Tsung-Yi Lin: A tri-axial classification of mental disorders in childhood. J. Child Psychol Psychiatr, 10:41, 1969.

200. Sandifer, M. G. Jr., Wilson, I. C., and Green, L.: The two-type theses of depressive disorders. Am J Psychiatr, 123:93, 1966.

201. Sargent, W.: The treatment of depressive states. Int J Neurol, 6:53, 1967.

202. Savage, C.: Lysergic acid diethylamide (LSD-25). A clinical-psychological study. Am J Psychiatr, 108:896, 1952.

203. Schiele, B. C., Vestre, N. D., and MacNaughton, D. V.: Treatment of hospitalized schizophrenics with trifluoperazine plus tranylcypromine. A double-blind controlled study. Compr Psychiatr, 4:66-72, 1963.

204. Schildkraut, J. J., and Kety, S. S.: Biogenic amines and emotion. Science, 156:21, 1967.

205. Schildkraut, J. J., Schanberg, S. M., Breese, G. R., and Kopin, I. J.: Norepinephrine metabolism and drugs used in the affective disorders: A possible mechanism of action. Am J Psychiatr, 124:54, 1967.

206. Schou, M.: Lithium in psychiatric therapy and prophylaxis. J Psychiatr Res, 6:67, 1968.

207. Seevers, M. H.: Morphine and ethanol physical dependence: A critique

of a hypothesis. Science 170:1113, 1970.

208. Sharpless, S. K.: Hypnotics and sedatives. I. Bartiturates. In Goodman, L., and Gilman, A. (Eds.): The Pharmacological Basis of Therapeutics, 4th ed. New York, Macmillan, 1970. pp. 98-120.

209. Shelton, J., and Hollister, L. E.: Simulated abuse of tybamate in man: Failure to demonstrate withdrawal reactions. JAMA, 199:338-340, 1967.

210. Shopsin, B., Kim, S. S., and Gershon, S.: A controlled study of lithium vs chlorpromazine in acute schizophrenics. Br J Psychiatr, 119:435, 1971.

211. Shopsin, B., Friedmann, R., and Gershon, S.: Lithium and leucocytosis. Clin Pharmacol Ther, 12:923, 1971.

212. Silverman, C.: The epidemiology of depression – A review. Am J Psychiatr, 124:43, 1968.

213. Singer, K., and Cheng, M. N.: Thiopropazate hydrochloride in persistent dyskinesia. Br Med J, 4:22, 1971.

214. Sjoquist, F.: Interaction between monoamine oxidase (MAO) inhibitors and other substances. Proc Roy Soc Med, 58:967, 1965.

215. Sjoquist, F., Hammer, W., Borga, O., and Azarnoff, D. L.: Pharmacological significance of the plasma level of monomethylated tricyclic antidepressants. In The Present Status of Psychotropic Drugs. Pharmacological and Clinical Aspects. Excerpta Medica Foundation, Amsterdam, 1969, p. 128.

216. Smith, L. H., Jr., and Becker, C. E.: Medical complications of heroin addiction. Calif Med, 115:42, 1971.

217. Stach, K., and Poldinger, W.: Strukturelle betrachutgen der psychopharmaka: Versuch einer korrelation von chemischer konstitution andclinischer wirkung. In Jucker, E. (Ed.): Progress in Drug Research. Basel, Birkhauser Verlag, 1966, pp. 129-190.

218. Stevenson, G.: Therapy – therapist. Ment Hyg, 35:529, 1951.

219. Stokes, P. E., Stoll, P. M., Shamoian, C. A., and Patton, M. J.: Efficacy of lithium as acute treatment of manic-depressive illness. Lancet 1:1319, 1971.

220. Stokes, J. W., Mendels, J., Secunda, S. K., and Dyson, W. L.: Lithium excretion and therapeutic response. J Nerv Ment Dis, 154:43, 1972.

221. Stolley, P. D., Becker, M. H., McEvilla, J. D., Lasagna, L., Gainor, M., and Sloane, L. M.: Drug prescribing and use in an American community. Ann Int Med, 76:537, 1972.

222. Tuthill, E. W., Overall, J. E., and Hollister, L. E.: Subjective correlates of clinically manifested anxiety and depression. Psychol Rep, 20:535, 1967.

223. Uhlenhuth, E. H., Rickels, K., Fisher, S., Park, L. C., Lipman, R. S., and Mock, J.: Drug, doctor's verbal attitude and clinic setting in the symptomatic response to pharmacotherapy. Psychopharmacologia, 9:392-418, 1966.

224. Usdin, E.: The assay of chlorpromazine and metabolites in blood, urine

and other tissues. CRC Crit Revs Clin Lab Sc, 2:347, 1971.
225. van der Kleijn, E., van Rossum, J. M., Muskens, E. T. J. M., and Rijntjes, N. V. M.: Pharmacokinetics of diazepam in dogs, mice and humans. Acta Pharmacol Toxicol, 29 (Supp. #3):109, 1971.
226. Van Praag, H. M., Schut, T., Dols, L., and Van Schilfgaarden, R.: Controlled trial of penfluridol in acute psychosis. Br Med J, 4:710, 1971.
227. Walter, C. J. S.: Clinical significance of plasma imipramine levels. Proc Roy Soc Med, 64:282, 1971.
228. Weil-Malherbe, H., and Szara, S. I.: The Biochemistry of Functional and Experimental Psychoses. Charles C Thomas, Springfield, Ill., 1971, pp. 53-91.
229. Weiss, G., Werry, J., Minde, K., Douglas, V., and Sykes, D.: Studies on the hyperactive child — V. The effects of dextroamphetamine and chlorpromazine on behavior and intellectual functioning. J Child Psychol Psychiatry, 9:145, 1968.
230. Werry, J. S.: The use of psychoactive drugs in children Ill Med J, 131:785, 1967.
231. Wheatley, D.: Comparative effects of propranolol and chlordiazepoxide in anxiety states. Br J Psychiatr, 115:1411-1412, 1969.
232. Williams, R. B., and Sherter, C.: Cardiac complications of tricyclic antidepressant therapy. Ann Int Med, 74:395, 1971.
233. Wilson, J. H. P., Donker, A. J. M., Van Der Hem, G. K., and Wientjes, J.: Peritoneal dialysis for lithium poisoning. Br Med J, 2:749, 1971.
234. Wilson, I. C., Prange, A. J., McClane, T. K., Rabon, A. M., and Lipton, M. A.: Thyroid-hormone enhancement of imipramine in nonretarded depressions. New Eng J Med, 282:1063-1067, 1970.
235. Wittenborn, J. R.: Psychiatric rating scales. New York, The Psychological Corporation, 1955.
236. Wittenborn, J. R., Plante, M., Burgess, F., and Maurer, H.: A comparison of imipramine, electroconvulsive therapy, and placebo in the treatment of depression. J Nerv Ment Dis, 135:131, 1962.
237. Zall, H., Therman, P. O. G., and Myers, J. M.: Lithium carbonate: A clinical study. Am J Psychiatr, 125:549, 1968.
238. Zeidenberg, P., Perel, J. M., Kanzler, M., Wharton, R. N., and Malitz, S.: Clinical and metabolic studies with imipramine in man. Am J Psychiatr, 127:1321, 1971.
239. Zeller, E. A., and Barsky, J.: In vivo inhibition of liver and brain monoamine oxidase by 1-isonicotinyl-2-isopropylhydrazine. Proc Soc Exp Biol Med, 81:459, 1952.
240. Zick, W. H.: Eine newartige behandlung der depression mit einer kombination von amitriptyline and protriptyline in der klinischen psychiatrie. Arzneim Forsch, 16:1616, 1966.
241. Zuckerman, M.: The development of an affect adjective check-list for the measurement of anxiety. J Consult Psychol, 24:457, 1960.

INDEX

compared with other drugs, 88-89
in endogenous depression, 88
interaction with chlorpromazine, 85
kinetics, 84-85
in retarded depression, 90
triiodothyronine and, 103
Inderal (propranolol)
insulin shock, 4
iproniazid (Marsilid), 5, 78
isocarboxazide (Marplan®), 77, 88, 97
isoniazid, 5

J

James-Lange hypothesis of anxiety, 112-113
jaundice, cholestatic
with phenothiazines, 50
with tricyclics, 106

K

Kemadrin® (procyclidine HCl)
Kraepelin, 1

L

Largatil (chlorpromazine)
levodopa (Larodopa), 20
aggravation of mental states, 58, 168-170
in depression, 105
levarterenol (l-norepinephrine), 52
Librium® (chlordiazepoxide)
limbic system 20
lithium carbonate, 29, 59, 170
discovery, 4
doses, dosage, 66-67
indications, 60-62
kinetics, 64-65
pharmacological action, 63
poisoning, 65
prophylactic use, 59-60
serum lithium levels, 67-68
side effects, 69-70
loxapine, 19
lysergic acid diethylamide (LSD), 5, 168
in depression, 104

M

Majeptil (thioproperazine)
manic-depressive psychosis, 56
antipsychotic drugs in, 65-66
diagnosis, 56-57
lithium treatment, 60-61
pathogenesis, 57
manic reaction, 29, 36
Marplan® (isocarboxazide)
Marsilid (iproniazid)
Mellaril® (thioridazine)
mental deficiency, 150-151
mepazine (Pacatal®), 26-27
meperidine (Demerol®), 4, 105
meprobamate (Miltown, Equanil®), 120, 134, 161
abuse, 159-161
combined with other drugs, 90, 94
compared with other drugs, 124-126
kinetics, 121-122
mesoridazine (Serentil), 15-16, 33
methadone, 164-165
methaqualone (Quaalude, Parest, Sapor)
abuse, 161-162
methamphetamine (Desoxyn®), 77, 97
methylphenidate (Ritalin®), 77-78, 97
in hyperkinetic children, 144
inhibition of hydroxylating enzymes, 87
methysergide (Sansert®), 58
metiapine, 19
metranidazole (Flagyl®), 157
Metrazol® (pentylenetetrazole)
Miltown® (meprobamate)
minimal brain damage see hyperkinetic)
Minnesota Multiphasic Personality Inventory, 115
models, drug-induced, 167-170
depression, 58, 168
Parkinson's disease, 168
schizophrenia, 168-170
model psychosis, 5, 168-169
molindone, 19, 26-27
monoamine oxidase inhibitors, 78, 88-89, 98
discovery, 5
interactions with other drugs, 106-107